CONTROVERSIES IN OBSTETRIC ANAESTHESIA

Number Two

Edited by
BARBARA MORGAN

Edward Arnold
A division of Hodder & Stoughton
LONDON MELBOURNE AUCKLAND

© 1993 Hodder and Stoughton Publishers Limited

First published in Great Britain 1993

British Library Cataloguing in Publication Data

Controversies in Obstetric Anaesthesia.
No. 2
I. Morgan, Barbara
617.9682

ISBN 0-340-55738-9

Whilst the advice and information in this book is believed to be true
and accurate at the date of going to press, neither the author nor the
publisher can accept any legal responsibility or liability for any errors
or omissions that may be made. In particular (but without limiting
the generality of the preceding disclaimer) every effort has been made
to check drug dosages; however, it is still possible that errors have
been missed. Furthermore, dosage schedules are constantly being
revised and new side effects recognised. For these reasons the reader is
strongly urged to consult the drug companies' printed instructions
before administering any of the drugs recommended in this book.

Typeset in 11/12pt Linotron Baskerville by
Rowland Phototypesetting Limited, Bury St Edmunds, Suffolk.
Printed and bound in Great Britain for Edward Arnold,
a division of Hodder and Stoughton Limited, Mill Road,
Dunton Green, Sevenoaks, Kent TN13 2YA by
Biddles Limited, Guildford and King's Lynn.

Preface

Obstetric anaesthestists in their developing speciality are somewhat prone to strong opinions. Debates allow views to be thoroughly examined. Occasionally the debate can change some anaesthetists' view, but always it can stimulate discussion and, more importantly, thought and possibly clinical research studies. Each of the argued controversies on which this book is based were in front of an audience, itself committed to the subject.

Unfortunately the views of the audience are not included in the book but add to the liveliness of the debate on the day, and can at times prove more pesuasive than the speakers'. An overview of papers that have upheld or refuted some controversies since the publication of the first volume of *Controversies in Obstetric Anaesthesia* is added. Many controversies seem to be evergreen, allowing discussion to continue without too many facts being researched, and no resolution of the problems.

Old wives' tales and apocryphal anecdotes form a not insubstantial part of obstetrics and thus of obstetric anaesthesia. In time these will be replaced by well-conducted studies and the controversies will be resolved.

Meanwhile the real benefit of this publication will accrue to the mother and child, who have a more aware, interested and informed anaesthetist.

Barbara Morgan
1992

Contents

1

No-one needs more than 30% oxygen for general anaesthesia caesarean section

ARGUMENTS FOR: T. A. Thomas

The use of gaseous mixtures containing 50% oxygen during the initial stages of general anaesthesia for caesarean section is an established practice, with some 20 years of history behind it. It is so well established that it has become an institutional practice in most obstetric units in this country. Pregnant women are almost the only group of fit adult patients to receive, routinely, such a high inspired concentration of oxygen during general anaesthesia.

Let us begin by exploring the background to this singular practice. A number of problems face anaesthetists of caesarean section patients. The intimate relationship between mother and fetus allows rapid equilibration, across the placenta, of many of the drugs administered to the mother. The fetus will therefore achieve plasma levels of most anaesthetic, sedative and analgesic drugs that closely follow those of the mother. Unfortunately these two individuals need to be in very different states during caesarean section. The mother should be anaesthetised, paralysed and pain free whilst the fetus should be wide awake with full muscle tone and no respiratory depression at birth. The relaxing effect of volatile anaesthetic agents on uterine muscle is another complicating problem.

The history of our present compromise is of importance to our debate. The use of a thiopentone, nitrous oxide, oxygen and muscle relaxant technique of anaesthesia with intermittent positive pressure ventilation became the standard method of anaesthesia for caesarean section following work done in the late 1950s and early 1960s.[1,2,3] Improvements in the condition of the fetus and neonate delivered by caesarean section under general anaesthesia were reported when 50–66% oxygen was administered as part of the inhalational anaesthetic mixture.[4,5,6] However, an incidence of 2–6 % awareness during caesarean section under this type of general anaesthesia was also reported.[7,8] The definitive paper drawing together the various aspects of anaesthesia for caesarean section at that time was written by Donald Moir.[9] It was this paper which, probably more than any other, established the use of 50% oxygen/nitrous oxide mixtures during anaesthesia for caesarean section.

The apparent importance of this accumulation of evidence from the 1950s and 1960s is, however, misleading. All of the investigations were carried out with the obstetric patient in the supine position, although Marx employed left uterine displacement, and pre-dated the report from Jeffrey Selwyn Crawford[10] in which he showed the overwhelming importance of aortocaval compression in relation to the incidence of fetal hypoxia, acidosis and low Apgar scores. The earlier work was therefore carried out on a disadvantaged fetal and neonatal population in whom any increase in maternal PaO_2 was bound to produce improvement. The proper solution to the problem was not an increase in maternal PaO_2 but relief of aortocaval compression by the use of lateral tilt. It is likely therefore that, with the introduction of lateral tilt as an integral part of anaesthesia for caesarean section, the need for high inspired concentrations of oxygen to improve fetal well-being has disappeared.

In fact, it is possible that the use of high F_1O_2 may be associated with changes which have a deleterious effect on the fetus. Chronic exposure to high inspired concentrations of oxygen has been associated with a number of well-recognised changes including retrosternal discomfort, nausea and vomiting, paraesthesiae, joint pain, contracted visual fields, mental changes and, in the neonate, retrolental fibroplasia. Cardiorespiratory changes are, however, more rapidly established. They include a reduction in vital capacity, atalectasis, interference with carbon dioxide transport, decreased pulse rate, decreased cardiac output, peripheral vasoconstriction and a raised systemic blood pressure. These effects are mild but undesirable during caesarean section as they may hinder placental maternofetal exchange and will be made worse by any increase in sympathetic autonomic activity. A degree of sympathetic response is seen during most forms or levels of general anaesthesia, but the use of deeper levels of anaesthesia and high doses of analgesic agents depresses these responses. Neither deep anaesthesia nor large doses of opioid are suitable components of anaesthesia for caesarean section. Lightening of anaesthesia by the use of high inspired concentrations of oxygen also leads to a greater risk of awareness, reported as 2–6% in the 1960s and 1970s. When awareness occurs, it leads to profound maternal stress responses that are known to disadvantage the fetus.[11] Obviously awareness during hyperoxic, opioid-free general anaesthesia is the worst of all circumstances. It creates serious problems for both mother and baby and must be prevented at all costs.

The addition of one or other volatile anaesthetic agent, in various concentrations, to prevent awareness has been suggested since the late 1960s (Table 1.1). However, as late as 1985, Crawford and his colleagues reported[12] incidences of awareness and/or unpleasant dreams which varied between 1.6% and 9.6% and which were only abolished in a group of 129 patients when halothane 0.5% was included in the inspired anaesthetic mixture (Table 1.2). The most critical period for awareness during caesarean section is the time between induction of anaesthesia and delivery of the baby. Volatile anaesthetic agents will indeed prevent awareness during this time if high enough plasma and central nervous system concentrations are

Table 1.1

Workers	O$_2$%	Volatile %		MAC equivalent when inspired = alveolar concentration
		Anaesthetics		
Rorke *et al.* 1968	33	Ether		>1 ⎤ Probably not
	66	Methoxyflurane		>1 ⎦ achieved during pre-delivery period
	100			
Baraka 1970	20	Halothane 0.5		0.48–1.0
	33			
	50			
	100			
Moir 1970	30			0.64
	50	Halothane 0.5		>1
	50	Halothane 0.8		>1
	93			
	28	Cyclopropane 6.5		Average approx. 0.66
Marx and Mateo 1971	33			but difficult to
	66	Fluroxene	1.25	calculate with the
	97	Fluroxene	2.5	diversity of combination
Crawford *et al.* 1985	66	Trichlorethylene		0.2
				0.3
		Halothane		0.2 ⎱ Varies between
				0.3 ⎰ 0.5 to 1.0
				0.
				0.5

Table 1.2

	T_2	T_3	H_2	H_3	H_4	H_5
No. of patients	135	128	129	129	127	129
Awareness	7	1	9	3	2	0
Unpleasant dreams	6	0	4	3	0	0
Percent combined complications	9.6	0.8	10.1	4.7	1.6	0

established before the anaesthetic effects of the intravenous induction agent has worn off. It is difficult to achieve this objective reliably with the volatile agents. The wash-in/equilibration curves of these drugs show that a significant time will elapse from introduction of the agent to the attainment of either equilibration between alveolar and plasma levels or the production of adequate depth of anaesthesia. The rapidity of onset of anaesthesia is affected by the inspired concentration of the anaesthetic agent in question. A type of 'overpressure' approach can be adopted which entails the use of a concentration of up to 3 × MAC in the inspired mixture. Concentration gradients between alveolar, plasma and CNS tissue are greater than usual when using this approach and it is quite possible that uterine muscle will be exposed to levels of the volatile agents that will cause some depression.[13] If circulating plasma levels of volatile anaesthetic agents rise to MAC levels, uterine contractility is depressed and eventually the oxytocic response is also affected. Marx *et al.*[13] showed quite clearly that this effect is seen with human myometrium just as it is with animal uterine muscle.

What is required is an inhalational anaesthetic agent which has a swift onset of action because of rapid equilibration between alveolar, plasma and CNS tissue levels, produces analgesia and which has a minimal effect on the uterus and the fetus.

Nitrous oxide is such an agent. It has an extremely rapid onset of action, a rapid wash-in curve and rapid equilibration characteristics. In addition, its presence in an anaesthetic gaseous mixture will increase the rapidity of effectiveness of volatile agents by the second gas effect. The higher the concentration of nitrous oxide in the mixture, the greater that enhancement of volatile agent will be through the concentration effect. Nitrous oxide, unlike volatile anaesthetics, exerts a minimal depressant effect on uterine muscle and produces effective analgesia in a significant proportion of those receiving it. These effects are so desirable that inclusion of nitrous oxide in as high a concentration as possible in a general anaesthetic would seem to be very advantageous.

Perhaps we should, in the light of these properties and the limitations of the pre-1972 reports which damned nitrous oxide, reconsider its role in caesarean section general anaesthesia. The critical question to be answered is: does the use of a mixture of 33% oxygen and 67% nitrous oxide produce adverse effects on the fetus or neonate? Lawes and his colleagues[14] investigated this very point. Their study compared two groups of mothers and babies. In one group the mother undergoing caesarean section received a 50% oxygen/nitrous oxide mixture and in the other group, 33% oxygen and 67% nitrous oxide. They found no significant difference between the condition of the babies in their two groups (Table 1.3) and concluded that: 'It is our view that an increased concentration of nitrous oxide can be used without detriment to the neonate in the absence of severe fetal distress'.

At the other extreme, Bogod and his colleagues[15] studied the effect of increasing the inspired concentration of oxygen to 100%. They used as controls a group of women who received 50% oxygen/nitrous oxide with 0.5% halothane and compared them with groups who received 100% oxygen plus $1.5 \times$ MAC of either halothane, enflurane or isoflurane. They identified few significant differences between the groups and the increase in umbilical venous PO_2 which they comment on particularly, is not statistically significant when individual groups are compared with the controls. It must be remembered that umbilical venous PO_2 changes usually follow closely any changes in maternal arterial levels if placental function remains unchanged.[16] The mothers in the study groups (100% F_1O_2) presumably achieved PaO_2 levels nearly twice those of the control (50% F_1O_2) group so it is surprising that such a large increase in maternal PaO_2 was not accompanied by a similarly great rise in umbilical venous PO_2. Perhaps a change in placental function did occur which limited arterialisation of fetal blood in those control groups. It has been shown in previous reports that increasing maternal F_1O_2 over 60% is not associated with further increases in umbilical PO_2. It is conceivable that this limitation of effect is due to the cardiovascular effects of hyperoxia.

Bogod also measured blood loss at operation and compared pre- and post-operative haemoglobin levels. The results are somewhat equivocal but seem to indicate that the groups receiving 100% oxygen with $1-1.5 \times$ MAC of enflurane or isoflurane suffered a greater blood loss than the control group.

Given the results of these two recent publications, the advantages of increasing inspired oxygen concentrations remain controversial whilst the uterine depressant effects of volatile agents have been confirmed. The babies in both studies, none of whom were suffering from severe fetal distress pre-operatively, did well and required minimal resuscitation. It would seem that neither the use of 100% oxygen or a 33% oxygen mixture made any difference to neonatal outcome.

Perhaps the deciding factor to hold the balance in this matter is

Table 1.3 Comparison of outcome variables for 50% and 33% oxygen concentration groups

	Group A 50% oxygen ($n = 16$)	Group B 33% oxygen ($n = 19$)	Statistics	A–B	95% CI for diff.
Umbilical vein,					
Mean Po_2 (kPa)	3.9	3.7	$t = 0.6$, $P = 0.5$	1.5	-3.3–6.1
Mean Pco_2 (kPa)	6.2	6.2	$t = -0.1$, $P = 0.9$	-0.2	-5.3–4.8
Mean pH	7.30	7.31	$t = -0.9$, $P = 0.4$	-0.01	-0.05–2.02
Time to spontaneous ventilation (s)					
Median	12.5	10.0	$w = 2.09$, $P = 0.5$	2.5	-5–90
Range	5–180	2–240			
Apgar (minus colour): No. with scores 7 or 8					
1 min	7 (43%)	9 (47%)	$\chi^2 = 0.02$, $P = 0.9$	-4%	-37–29%
5 min	16 (100%)	17 (89%)	—		
Induction-delivery interval (min)					
Median	7.0	8.0	$w = 274$, $P = 0.7$	-1.0	-3.0–1.7
Range	5–12	2–20			
Uterine incision-delivery interval (s)					
Median	80.0	87.0	$w = 270$, $P = 0.6$	-7	-45–30
Range	15–240	30–480			

that of awareness. Much has been written about awareness in both the medical and lay press. Many claim that patients who are aware feel no pain. Certainly Tunstall, in his original report[17] of use of the 'isolated arm' technique, gives no suggestion that patients were in pain and a more recent report has made similar observations, although it did record a small number of instances of 'unpleasant recall'.[18] However, reports in the lay press, often relating to cases being brought to the courts, have been very different. They have reported 'agonising pain' during anaesthesia. The press sensationalism received corroboration from an editorial in the BJA of 1979.[19] It comprised 'the unedited recollections of a medically qualified lady who experienced a Caesarean section under general anaesthesia which was insufficient to prevent awareness during part of the procedure'. She wrote:

> I understood my predicament. I was lying there intubated, covered in green towels, my abdomen split open and strange people delving inside me. My first reaction to this was an irrational surge of fear and panic.

She goes on to say:

> The closest parallel I can think of is of being in a coffin having been buried alive . . . I remained in this state of mind . . . continuously filled with fear, listening to every word and every sound in the theatre, quite compos mentis, fully appreciating my position. One pint of beer would have dulled my mind more than the anaesthetic.
>
> Every sensation which intruded into my emptiness seemed to startle me. I couldn't see so I had absolutely no warning of what was coming. Of course I heard the baby crying. I thought, there's a baby crying. How odd in theatre. Oh, it's my baby. And I am ashamed to say I felt absolutely no emotion at this, such was my fear and terror.
>
> Very suddenly I had the most horrible sensation, down the back of my throat, as of rough fingers marching down my throat . . . Oh, it's only the nasogastric tube.

After recording some other sensations she continued:

> There came three rough stripes across my abdomen. Almost before the third stripe had finished it was followed by the pain, as suddenly as though I had been stabbed. I thought Oh no, this isn't supposed to happen, you're not supposed to feel the pain. The nearest comparison would be the pain of a tooth pulled without anaesthetic when the drill hits a nerve. Multiply this pain so that the area involved would equal a thumb print and pour a steady stream of molten lead into it. If you imagine the effect of a too hot pan moved

from a cooker to a plastic surface, that is what the pain was doing to my non-existent body, searing, melting, pressing me into the table, and hurting me terribly.

I would pay a very high price to prevent that happening to any of my patients. At present I believe that the use of 'anaesthetic' concentrations of 70% nitrous oxide with 30% oxygen assists substantially in that prevention. The reported disadvantages of using such concentrations are largely historical and have not been confirmed using current anaesthetic techniques. Much more work needs to be done before we abandon such a beneficial gaseous anaesthetic mixture.

* *

ARGUMENTS AGAINST: D. Bogod

The increasing acceptability of epidural and spinal anaesthesia amongst mothers, anaesthetists and obstetricians has recently resulted in a decrease in the proportion of caesarean sections being performed under general anaesthesia. In some centres in the UK, this trend is now so well established that general anaesthesia is the exception rather than the rule, even for emergency procedures. This change of practice is to be welcomed, reducing as it does the complications of gastric aspiration, failed intubation, painful awareness and fetal sedation, which have always made a substantial contribution to maternal and fetal mortality and morbidity. There will, however, continue to be a requirement for general anaesthesia in some cases and, as the technique will be more rarely used, it becomes increasingly important that trainees learning obstetric anaesthesia are correctly instructed to compensate for the reduction in practical experience.

Modern practice has been based upon the work of Moir,[9] who first suggested the use of 0.5% halothane to supplement a mixture of 50% nitrous oxide and 50% oxygen in the post-induction, pre-delivery period. Recently, concern about awareness has resulted in some anaesthetists advocating a reduction in the inspired concentration of oxygen to 30% (F_IO_2 0.3). They have been encouraged in this view by the wide availability of pulse oximetry, which has shown that mothers ventilated with this mixture do not become hypoxic—the fear of hypoxia resulting from the imposition of positive pressure ventilation upon the already increased ventilation–perfusion mismatch of the pregnant patient was certainly one of the concerns that led to the adoption of 50% oxygen as the standard. But the mother is not the only patient under our care during caesarean section; the fetus demands our consideration also and, as I will argue, is short-changed when we use less than 50% oxygen for caesarean section under general anaesthesia.

In arguing my case, I shall be drawing upon the results of several studies which examine the effect of different maternal inspired oxygen concentrations upon fetal well-being. Degree of asphyxia in the immediate pre-delivery period has traditionally been assessed by the one-minute Apgar score,[20] and this is the measure employed by the authors to whose work I will refer. Although detailed neuro-behavioural tests, such as the Brazelton score,[21] may be more sensitive in detecting the effects of perinatal asphyxia, their use in this particular field has been scanty.

Dr Trevor Thomas, my respected opponent in this debate, has dismissed the low Apgar scores found by other workers in babies whose mothers received 70% nitrous oxide during caesarean section.[14] He says: 'The physical findings of apnoea, cyanosis, bradycardia and hypotonus implicit in an Apgar score of 3 do not reflect the known pharmacological properties of nitrous oxide in the neonate'. Of course they do not, just as the 'jactitations' seen by earlier anaesthetists in dental patients were not a side effect of the 100% nitrous oxide that they received. The fits, for that was what they were, were the result of hypoxia and so were the low Apgar scores that Dr Thomas treats in such a dismissive fashion. I hope to show that those who use 30% oxygen for caesarean section may be failing in one of the prime duties of the anaesthetist—the prevention of hypoxia.

It will be evident to the reader that my argument will be based on the premise that a baby born to a mother who is ventilated with 30% oxygen suffers a period of relative hypoxia during caesarean delivery. What is the evidence for this?

We certainly have little to be complacent about when we consider the state of the baby delivered by caesarean section under general anaesthesia. Even in elective cases, where delivery of a healthy, lively baby is anticipated, low Apgar scores at one minute are often found, suggesting a brief period of asphyxia immediately prior to delivery. This is graphically illustrated by a large retrospective study from South Wales[22] which looked at a cohort of babies presenting by the vertex without fetal distress and with a birth weight greater than 2.5 kg—healthy fetuses, in fact (Table 1.4). When delivered vaginally, 13% had a one-minute Apgar score of 4–7 and only 2% a score of 3 or less. When delivered by elective general anaesthetic caesarean section, for reasons unrelated to the well-being of the fetus, these percentages increased to 28% and 5% respectively.

These findings are even borne out by a study conducted by Dr Thomas, my opponent in this debate.[14] Of his 35 patients delivered by caesarean section, none with fetal distress, 55% had an Apgar-minus-colour score (maximum 8) of 6 or less, a score that Selwyn

Crawford[23] described as indicative of moderate asphyxia (Table 1.4). Why should this disparity exist, where a substantial number of babies are delivered in less than ideal condition, despite there being no evidence of fetoplacental problems prior to delivery? These poor results must be due to factors related directly to caesarean delivery which are not present during vaginal delivery.

Table 1.4   Apgar scores of unstressed neonates at vaginal delivery and caesarean section

	1-minute Apgar score		
	8–10	*4–7*	*<4*
Vaginal	85%	13%	2%
GA caesarean section	67%	28%	5%
	(Murphy, Dauncey, *et al. Anaesthesia* 1984; **39**: 760)		
	1-minute Apgar-minus-colour score (max. 8)		
	7–8	*<7*	
GA caesarean section	45%	55%	
	(Lawes, Newman, *et al. Br J Anaesth* 1988; **61**: 250)		

The first of these factors is evident enough. Caesarean section patients are delivered under the effect of general anaesthesia. Lipid-soluble anaesthetic drugs, whether administered intravenously or by inhalation, will readily cross the placenta, resulting in neonatal sedation. This will directly affect the Apgar score by reducing tone and reflex irritability and indirectly by depressing respiration, thus adversely affecting oxygenation.

The second factor which compromises the baby delivered by caesarean section is the effect of general anaesthesia upon uterine blood flow and placental perfusion. Despite the use of lateral tilt in these patients, the myocardial depressant effect of inhalational anaesthetic agents will enhance the effect of aortocaval compression. Compression of the inferior vena cava will decrease the venous return to the heart and hence cardiac output. Partial obstruction of the abdominal aorta will further reduce flow through the uterine arteries. This situation will be worsened by uterine artery vasoconstriction resulting from endogenous catecholamine release during endotracheal intubation and light anaesthesia.

A further factor to be taken into account is the period of greatly decreased placental flow which commences when the uterus is incised. From this point until the baby is delivered from the amniotic sac, its supply of oxygen is markedly curtailed and its own oxygen reserves become rapidly depleted.[24]

Finally, the baby born by caesarean section is deprived of the compressive forces that occur during vaginal delivery. These forces are beneficial in that they squeeze the thoracic cage, thus tending to reduce lung water and therefore improve the efficiency of gas exchange in the lungs from the first breath.[25]

To summarise, it would perhaps be over-fanciful to describe the neonate delivered by caesarean section under general anaesthesia as being sedated, shocked, asphyxiated and suffering from pulmonary oedema, but each of these conditions is represented to some degree in the situations described above. It is hardly surprising that unexpectedly low Apgar scores are found in these circumstances!

It would seem prudent to prepare the neonate for this traumatic episode by increasing its oxygen reserves as much as possible, the equivalent of pre-oxygenation in an adult patient. Successful pre-oxygenation of the fetus will be reflected in an umbilical vein PO_2 that is significantly higher than that of babies delivered vaginally to mothers breathing room air. Before I go on to discuss how this pre-oxygenation may be best achieved, can it be demonstrated that the normoxic fetus is disadvantaged during the stresses of caesarean birth?

The umbilical vein PO_2 following normal, vertex vaginal delivery is variously reported as lying between 2.8 and 4.0 kPa.[26,27,28] Several studies have looked at varying inspired oxygen concentrations during elective caesarean section and this figure is consistently achieved by the use of a maternal F_IO_2 of around 0.3 (Table 1.5). For example, in Rorke's study[4] the babies born to the 33% oxygen group had a mean umbilical vein PO_2 of 3.8 kPa. This was raised to 5.2 kPa in the mothers who received 66% oxygen. In Moir's classic paper[9] 35% of the babies born to the normoxic group (33% inspired oxygen) had an Apgar score of 4–7 and 10% a score of 3 or less. In the hyperoxic group (50% inspired oxygen), these figures were 8% and 3% respectively. Gertie Marx demonstrated similar results[5]—in her normoxic babies (umbilical vein PO_2 3.9 kPa, F_IO_2 30%), 12 out of 25 had a one minute Apgar score of 7 or less, compared to only four out of 25 in the group with an umbilical vein PO_2 of 4.6 kPa, whose mothers

Table 1.5 Umbilical vein PO_2 and maternal F_IO_2 at delivery

Type of delivery	F_IO_2	Umbilical vein PO_2 (kPa)
Vertex vaginal	0.21	2.8–4.0
Elective GA caesarean section:		
Rorke, Davey and DuToit	0.33	3.8
Marx and Mateo	0.30	3.9
Baraka	0.33	3.9
Lawes, Newman, *et al.*	0.33	3.7

were ventilated with 65% oxygen. Marx goes on to point out that the babies from her hyperoxic group would have a 25% greater oxygen reserve than those from the normoxic group. This is achieved by replacement of nitrogen stores with oxygen in the same way that pre-oxygenation increases the reserve of the mother.

It might be supposed that babies delivered by caesarean section would fare better when regional anaesthesia was used, but Ramanathan has shown that the normoxic baby is still compromised even in these circumstances.[16] In his study, mothers breathing room air had babies with a mean umbilical vein PO_2 of 3.7 kPa and a base deficit of 4.5 mmol/l. This base deficit was reduced to 1.2 mmol/l in babies with an umbilical vein PO_2 of 4.7 kPa whose mothers breathed 47% oxygen.

There can be no doubt that these figures demonstrate that the hyperoxygenated baby emerges in a better state than its normoxic counterpart. The study by Dr Thomas and his colleagues[14] set out to disprove this hypothesis, but failed at the first obstacle; despite the use of 50% oxygen, their high-oxygen group did *not* deliver hyperoxygenated babies. In fact, the mean PO_2 of the babies in this group was only 3.9 kPa, well within the normoxic range, compared to 5.2 kPa in Rorke's study, 4.6 kPa in Gertie Marx's group, and 4.9 kPa in a recently published paper from Cardiff.[29] It is a matter for conjecture why this disparity occurs, but it does negate the conclusion of the paper, that the use of a high maternal F_IO_2 is of no benefit to the baby—it *is* of benefit, but only when it results in neonatal hyperoxygenation.

All of the work mentioned so far has one thing in common—none of the caesarean sections were performed for fetal distress, usually one of the commonest indications for this procedure. This is because the studies were confined to Selwyn Crawford's 'ideal clinical cases', in order to minimise any extraneous differences between the patients, thus making comparison between the groups easier. In the real world, however, not only do a lot of patients have fetoplacental units that are far from ideal, but in this age of regional anaesthesia for elective surgery, it is patients with fetal distress who probably make up the largest group undergoing general anaesthetic caesarean section. If 50% oxygen is needed to hyperoxygenate the well-perfused fetus, how much more is needed for the fetus whose blood supply is compromised by pre-eclampsia, cord compression or abruption?

Piggott *et al*. have attempted to answer this question by comparing the use of 50% and 100% oxygen in both elective and emergency procedures.[29] In all groups, the depth of anaesthesia was controlled by adding isoflurane so that the inspired mixture delivered 1.5 MAC for the first five minutes and 1.0 MAC thereafter until delivery (Table 1.6). As might be predicted from the studies mentioned earlier, in the

Table 1.6 Mean umbilical vein pO_2 (kPa) in patients undergoing GA Caesarean section with varying inspired oxygen concentration ($\pm$SD). Piggott *et al. Br J Anaesth* 1990

	50% oxygen	100% oxygen	
Elective group	4.9 (1.0)	5.8 (1.8)	N.S.
Emergency group	4.0 (1.2)	5.0 (1.8)	p<0.01

elective patients the mean umbilical vein PO_2 in the 50% group was in the hyperoxic range that has already been demonstrated as being beneficial (4.9 kPa). The use of 100% oxygen raised this figure to 5.8 kPa, but this difference was not statistically significant. A different story emerges from the patients undergoing emergency caesarean section, many for fetal distress. In this group, with compromised placental perfusion, the mean umbilical vein PO_2 was only 4.0 kPa when 50% oxygen was used. Hence, despite the use of an inspired oxygen concentration regarded by Dr Thomas as unnecessarily high, the babies remain normoxic and disadvantaged. When the inspired oxygen concentration was increased to 100%, however, the umbilical vein PO_2 rose to 5.0 kPa, well into the hyperoxygenated range.

Having established the need for 100% oxygen to achieve hyperoxygenation in the distressed fetus, the study goes on to examine whether the same benefits can be demonstrated for this group as for the patients of other workers who received 50% oxygen during elective caesarean section. Figure 1.1 shows the one-minute Apgar scores for the babies delivered by emergency caesarean section. There is an obvious trend towards higher scores in the 100% oxygen group,

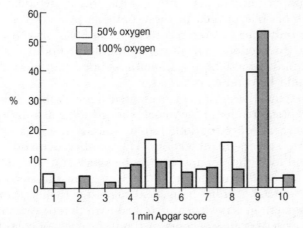

Fig. 1.1 One-minute Apgar scores of patients undergoing emergency GA caesarean section with varying inspired oxygen concentration (from Piggott *et al. British Journal of Anaesthesia* 1990)

although this does not reach statistical significance. When the degree of resuscitation deemed necessary by the attending paediatrician was examined, however, a significant difference was seen (Fig. 1.2). A larger number of babies from the 100% oxygen group needed airway suction only, and fewer needed oxygen insufflation, bagging on a mask or intubation.

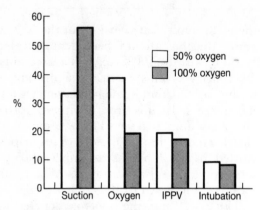

Fig. 1.2 Neonatal resuscitation required following GA caesarean section with varying inspired oxygen concentration (from Piggott *et al. British Journal of Anaesthesia* 1990)

These results, although not as conclusive as those confirming the benefits of 50% over 30% oxygen for elective caesarean section, are certainly food for thought when dealing with a patient who needs a 'crash' procedure for severe fetal distress; they also help to confirm the general hypothesis that hyperoxygenated fetuses do better. Perhaps more importantly in the context of the present debate, they show that the use of 50% oxygen in these patients produced a normoxic fetus. I can only guess at the results of using 30% oxygen for emergency caesarean section—for, in the light of these findings, the ethics of such a study would be questionable—but I am sure that fetal hypoxia would be commonly found.

I am sure that the argument presented above will convince even the most sceptical reader of the benefits to the fetus of a high inspired maternal oxygen concentration, but of course the fetus is not our only concern at caesarean section. The mother demands our due consideration also and, for my case to be successful, I must demonstrate that she suffers no detrimental effect from the steps taken to improve the outcome for her baby. As I suggested earlier, the question of hyperoxygenation is inextricably linked with that of awareness, and this in turn arises because of concern about the effect of volatile agents upon uterine contractility. These factors will be individually considered.

Awareness

The reduction or omission of nitrous oxide from an anaesthetic mixture has two consequences upon anaesthetic depth. Firstly, the MAC value of the mixture is directly lowered; secondly, the second gas effect, which speeds uptake of the volatile agent, is reduced or lost.

Nitrous oxide is, of course, a relatively weak anaesthetic agent with a MAC of approximately 100%. This means that increasing the inspired nitrous oxide concentration from 50% to 70% would result in a rise of only 0.2 MAC in the anaesthetic mixture, assuming that the agents in the mixture have an additive effect upon the MAC value. Even the use of 100% oxygen for emergency procedures would only reduce the potency of the anaesthetic by 0.5 MAC, when compared to a 50/50 regime.

It is upon the argument of awareness that the 30% nitrous oxide lobby base their case, but an increase in MAC value of 0.2 seems a negligible benefit when weighed against the increased neonatal morbidity described above. Moir[9] did not find a single case of painful awareness in his patients who received 50% nitrous oxide supplemented by 0.5% halothane, and he has subsequently been vindicated by other workers.[30,31,32] I have yet to hear of a patient suffering from painful awareness in whom this technique was correctly used; a recent case[33] probably resulted from the volatile agent being discontinued immediately after delivery, a practice which should be avoided.

If a more potent anaesthetic is desired, it would seem more efficacious to increase the concentration of volatile agent, rather than to decrease the oxygen. Thus, 0.2 MAC may be gained by changing the halothane concentration from 0.5% to 0.65%; an increase to 0.875% adds 0.5 MAC, and compensates for the loss of 50% nitrous oxide in emergency patients.

The loss of the second gas effect means that the uptake of volatile agent will be slowed; this will lead to an increased risk of awareness in the vital first few minutes of the procedure, after the intravenous induction agent has been redistributed from CNS tissue and before the alveolar concentration of volatile agent has reached anaesthetic levels. This can be compensated for by using a higher inspired concentration of agent in the first few minutes after induction—the so-called 'overpressure' technique. Thus, in the 100% oxygen group in the Cardiff study[29], 1.8% isoflurane was administered for five minutes, reducing to 1.2% thereafter; this is equipotent to 1.125% halothane reducing to 0.75%. Four out of the 200 patients in the Cardiff study reported dreaming when questioned post-operatively, divided equally between the 50% and 100% oxygen groups. In no case was the experience associated with pain.

In summary, there is no evidence that the correct use of 50% nitrous oxide supplemented by 0.7 MAC of a volatile agent is associated with a significant incidence of painful awareness. Even if it were, the potency of the anaesthetic could be best enhanced by increasing the concentration of volatile agent. Even the total absence of nitrous oxide can be compensated for by using more volatile agent, with a further increase in concentration in the first five minutes to make up for the loss of the second gas effect. The only question that remains to be addressed is whether uterine tone, and hence blood loss, is adversely affected by the increase in volatile agent.

Uterine tone

Most of the work on uterine contractility and volatile anaesthetic agents has been done with halothane, but enflurane and isoflurane have been shown to have a similar effect upon the uterus at equi-MAC concentrations, so the findings can be justifiably extrapolated to the more recently introduced agents.

Experiments with isolated rat myometrium[34] show that 0.65% halothane (equivalent to 1% isoflurane) reduces the resting tone of the muscle and 0.8% halothane (1.3% isoflurane) affects the tension developed during spontaneous contractions. These results show a noticeable effect *in vitro* of quite low concentrations of volatile agents, and might suggest that the clinical concentrations described above would indeed reduce the tone of the myometrium, leading to increased blood loss. Other workers have shown, however, that the sensitivity of the human uterus to volatile agents is considerably reduced in pregnancy, possibly by as much as a factor of 10.[35] A consistent finding in these *in vitro* studies is the rapid recovery of myometrial tone (within 2–5 minutes) following withdrawal of halothane.

The duration between induction and delivery is also an important consideration when evaluating the effect of the volatile agent. The uterus at term has a very high blood flow, and comes under the category of a 'vessel-rich' organ. The concentration of volatile agent reaching it via the uterine arteries will therefore rapidly equilibrate with the alveolus. But, of course, the alveolar concentration itself needs time to approach the inspired concentration, and this is a major factor even with the modern low-solubility volatile agents. In general, it has been shown that arterial blood halothane levels corresponding to an alveolar concentration as high as 0.8 MAC, while affecting peak contractions, have little effect on resting myometrial tone and do not diminish the effect of oxytocic drugs.[13] To achieve this sort of alveolar concentration within 20 minutes of induction would require an inspired level of 1.1% halothane (equivalent to 1.7% isoflurane). Even if no nitrous oxide were used, as in the Cardiff study, the maximum concentration of isoflurane required would only be 1.8% and this would reduce to 1.2% after five minutes. As the mean induction–delivery interval in that study was 11 minutes, it would be surprising if any adverse effects upon uterine contractility were seen. Although a direct assessment of the uterus was not made, blood loss was estimated by comparing the haemoglobin concentration and haematocrit 48 hours post-delivery with pre-operative levels (Table 1.7). It can be seen that the change was actually slightly less in the 100% oxygen group, although this result was not statistically significant.

Table 1.7 Mean (±SD) post-operative changes in haemoglobin concentration and haematocrit following GA Caesarean section with varying inspired oxygen concentration. Piggott *et al. Br J Anaesth* 1990

	50% oxygen	100% oxygen
Fall in Hb (g/dl) at 48 hours	1.19 (2.35)	1.10 (1.30)
Fall in Hct (%) at 48 hours	3.18 (5.57)	2.91 (3.78)

It would seem, therefore, that even these high levels of volatile agent do not have a measurable effect upon blood loss, as long as the induction–delivery interval is not unduly prolonged. Certainly, if at any time it was shown that the use of 50% nitrous oxide and 0.5% halothane was associated with an unacceptable level of awareness (which, as I have argued, is not yet the case) then the simple remedy of a 25% increase in the concentration of volatile agent would safely achieve the same effect as dropping the inspired oxygen concentration to 30%.

Conclusion

The argument in favour of 30% oxygen for caesarean section under general anaesthesia has been gaining support for some years. In part, this has been due to fears regarding awareness (or, more accurately, fears regarding litigation arising from awareness, as I am sure the incidence of this complication has fallen dramatically in the last 20 years since the routine use of potent volatile agents). Regrettably, the other main stimulus of this trend is the erroneous assumption that 50% oxygen was used to prevent maternal desaturation.

I hope that I have convincingly demonstrated the following:

1 That the stresses imposed by caesarean delivery result in a variable period of intrapartum fetal hypoxia, for which the normoxic fetus is ill prepared.
2 That the use of 30% oxygen fails to hyperoxygenate the fetus in preparation for this traumatic period.
3 That 50% oxygen will provide fetal pre-oxygenation in the presence of a well-perfused fetoplacental unit, but as much as 100% oxygen may be needed when pathology such as pre-eclampsia, cord compression or abruption is present.

4   That awareness can be prevented by the use of a potent volatile agent, without adversely affecting uterine contractility or blood loss.

In conclusion, I would strongly oppose the motion and would instead say that no *mother* needs more than 30% oxygen, but the baby does!

REFERENCES

1.   Hodges RJH, Bennett JR, Tunstall ME, Knight RF. General anaesthesia for operative obstetrics. *British Journal of Anaesthesia* 1959; **31:** 152.

2.   Hodges RJH, Tunstall ME. Choice of anaesthetic and its influence on perinatal mortality in caesarean section. *British Journal of Anaesthesia* 1961; **33:** 572.

3.   Crawford JS. Anaesthesia for caesarean section: a proposed method of evaluation with analysis of a technique. *British Journal of Anaesthesia* 1962; **34:** 179.

4.   Rorke MJ, Davey DA, Dutoit HJ. Fetal oxygenation during caesarean section. *Anaesthesia* 1968; **23:** 585.

5.   Marx GF, Mateo CV. Effects of different oxygen concentrations during general anaesthesia for elective caesarean section. *Canadian Anaesthetists Society Journal* 1971; **18:** 587.

6.   Baraka A. Correlation between maternal and fetal PO_2 and PCO_2 during caesarean section. *British Journal of Anaesthesia* 1970; **42:** 434.

7.   Heartridge VB, Wilson RB. Balanced anaesthesia for caesarean section. *American Journal of Obstetrics and Gynecology* 1963; **85:** 619.

8.   Wilson J, Turner DJ. Awareness during caesarean section under general anaesthesia. *British Medical Journal* 1969; **1:** 280.

9.   Moir DD. Anaesthesia for caesarean section: an evaluation of a method using low concentrations of halothane and 50% oxygen. *British Journal of Anaesthesia* 1970; **42:** 136.

10. Crawford JS, Burton M, Davies P. Time and lateral tilt at caesarean section. *British Journal of Anaesthesia* 1972; **44:** 477.

11. Morishima HO, Pederson H, Finster M. Influence of maternal psychological stress on the fetus. *American Journal of Obstetrics and Gynecology* 1978; **131:** 286.

12. Crawford JS, Lewis M, Davies P. Maternal and neonatal responses related to the volatile agent used to maintain anaesthesia at caesarean section. *British Journal of Anaesthesia* 1985; **57:** 482–7.

13. Marx GF, Kim YI, Lin C-C, Halevy S, Shulman H. Postpartum uterine pressures under halothane or enflurane anaesthesia. *Obstetrics and Gynecology* 1978; **51:** 695–8.

14. Lawes EG, Newman B, Campbell MJ, Irwin M, Dolenska S, Thomas TA. Maternal inspired oxygen concentration and neonatal status for caesarean section and general anaesthesia. *British Journal of Anaesthesia* 1988; **61:** 250.

15. Bogod DG, Rosen M, Rees GAD. Maximum F_1O_2 during caesarean section. *British Journal of Anaesthesia* 1988; **61:** 255.
16. Ramanathan S, Shamala G, Arismendy J, Chalon J, Turndorf H. Oxygen transfer from mother to fetus during caesarean section under epidural anaesthesia. *Anesthesia and Analgesia* 1982; **61:** 576–81.
17. Tunstall ME. Detecting wakefulness during general anaesthesia for caesarean section. *British Medical Journal* 1977; **1:** 1321.
18. Bogod DG, Orton JK, Yau HN, Oh TE. Detecting awareness during general anaesthetic caesarean section. *Anaesthesia* 1990; **45:** 279–84.
19. Editorial. On being aware. *British Journal of Anaesthesia* 1979; **51:** 711–12.
20. Apgar V. A proposal for a new method of evaluation of the newborn infant. *Current Research in Anesthesia* 1953; **32:** 260.
21. Brazelton TB. Neonatal behavioral assessment scale. In: *Clinics in developmental medicine*, vol. 50. Philadelphia: Lippincot, 1973.
22. Murphy JF, Dauncey M, Rees GAD, Rosen M, Gray OP. Obstetric analgesia, anaesthesia and the Apgar score. *Anaesthesia* 1984; **39:** 760.
23. Crawford JS. *Principles and practice of obstetric anaesthesia*. 4th edn. Oxford: Blackwell Scientific Publications, 1978.
24. Crawford JS, James FM, Davies P, Crawley M. A further study of general anaesthesia for caesarean section. *British Journal of Anaesthesia* 1976; **47:** 482.
25. Klein M. Asphyxia neonatorum caused by foaming. *Lancet* 1972; **1:** 1089.
26. Gare DJ, Shime J, Paul WM, Hoskins M. Oxygen administration during labor. *American Journal of Obstetrics and Gynecology* 1969; **105:** 954.
27. McClure JH, James JM. Oxygen administration to the mother and its relation to blood oxygen in the newborn infant. *American Journal of Obstetrics and Gynecology* 1960; **80:** 554.
28. Vasicka A, Quilligan EJ, Aznar R, Lipsitz PJ, Bloor BM. Oxygen tension in maternal and fetal blood, amniotic fluid, and cerebrospinal fluid of the mother and the baby. *American Journal of Obstetrics and Gynecology* 1960; **79:** 1041.
29. Piggott SE, Bogod DG, Rosen M, Rees GAD, Harmer M. Isoflurane with either 100% oxygen or 50% nitrous oxide in oxygen for caesarean section. *British Journal of Anaesthesia* 1990; **65:** 325.
30. Abboud TK, Kim SH, Henriksen EH, Chen T, Eisenman R, Levinson G, Shnider SM. Comparative maternal and neonatal effects of halothane and enflurane for caesarean section. *Acta Anaesth Scand* 1985; **29:** 663.
31. Warren TM, Datta S, Ostheimer GW, Naulty JS, Weiss JB, Morrison JA. Comparison of the maternal and neonatal effects of halothane, enflurane and isoflurane for caesarean delivery. *Anesthesia and Analgesia* 1983; **62:** 516.
32. Morgan BM, Aulakh JM, Barker JP, Goroszeniuk T, Trojanowski A. Anaesthesia for caesarean section: a medical audit of junior anaesthetic staff practice. *British Journal of Anaesthesia* 1983; **55:** 885.
33. Brahams D. Caesarean section: pain and awareness without negligence. *Anaesthesia* 1990; **45:** 161.

34. Naftalin NJ, Phear WPC, Goldberg AH. Halothane and isometric contractions of isolated pregnant rat myometrium. *Anesthesiology* 1975; **42:** 458.
35. McDonald-Gibson WJ. The influence of halothane on isolated human uterine muscle. *Journal of Obstetrics and Gynaecology of the British Commonwealth* 1969; **76:** 362.

2

Pre-loading prior to regional block is an old wives' tale

ARGUMENTS FOR: D. Scott

'Pre-loading', meaning the intravenous administration of fluid, either as an electrolyte solution or as a colloid, just before and during the onset of epidural blockade to prevent the development of hypotension, is standard practice for caesarean section performed under epidural or spinal anaesthesia. Indeed, many would consider it mandatory. This in spite of the fact that the logic behind it is faulty, the evidence for efficacy minimal and the failure rate high.

The cardiovascular status of the patient at the end of pregnancy differs from the non-pregnant state quite significantly in that:

- The cardiac output is increased by 1–2 l/min.
- The blood volume is increased by about 1 litre.
- The mean arterial pressure is decreased by 5–10 mmHg. A systolic pressure less than 100 mmHg is not uncommon, though during anaesthesia many anaesthetists would consider this abnormal and treatable. The increased cardiac output and decreased pressure mean that the peripheral resistance is much lower than in the non-pregnant.
- The heart rate increases by about 5 beats/min.
- The uterine blood flow is of the order of 500 ml/min.
- Caval occlusion can occur, especially when lying supine.[1] The overall effect of this depends upon the adequacy of the collateral venous circulation returning blood to the heart.[2] A large number of mothers do not exhibit any fall in arterial pressure even though the venous return (and therefore the cardiac output) is reduced. The arterial pressure is maintained by peripheral vasoconstriction. Although apparently normal clinically, they can suffer rapid

and marked hypotension in response to vasodilation. It is important to remember that caval occlusion can only be totally relieved
by assuming a full lateral position. Tilting with a wedge may
relieve it but is not guaranteed to do so.

- Aortic compression, also in the supine position, may lower arterial
  pressure in the lower part of the body while raising it in the upper
  body.[3] Uterine blood flow may decrease markedly.
- At delivery, aortocaval compression is totally relieved and uterine
  blood flow decreases dramatically. These can greatly augment
  venous return and cardiac output.
- Conversely, blood loss, sometimes severe, can occur.

Epidural blockade in **non-pregnant** patients causes vasodilation,
the degree being dependent upon the extent of the block. Anaesthesia
to the mid-thoracic dermatomes leads to vasodilation in the lower
body and a reflex vasoconstriction in the upper body. If the upper
thoracic dermatomes (T1–5) are included, the sympathetic output to
the heart is blocked, leading to bradycardia and a degree of negative
inotropism, with a resulting decrease in cardiac output of 10–15%.
In spite of these changes, hypotension due to the epidural blockade
alone is relatively uncommon even with high blocks.[4]

Epidural blockade in **late pregnancy**, however, is commonly associated with hypotension because it not only 'reveals' those patients
maintaining their arterial pressure in spite of caval occlusion, it can
also trigger vasovagal overactivity. The rapid appearance of hypotension, bradycardia and nausea are diagnostic of a vasovagal attack. In
severe cases, a faint can occur with a transient cardiac standstill
lasting a few seconds.

It can easily be seen that the situation is complex and the anaesthetist must monitor the patient assiduously and be prepared to react
without delay. Maintaining rapport with the patient is one of the best
ways of monitoring, and will frequently diagnose the early signs of
vagal overactivity.

Of the many cardiovascular changes that are occurring, however,
loss of fluid is not amongst them. How then can the administration
of fluid prevent hypotension, remembering that the essential trigger
to any decrease in arterial pressure is vasodilation? Arterial pressure
is the product of cardiac output and peripheral resistance. Fluids,
therefore, can only be effective if they increase the output, which
still leaves the primary cause of the hypotension, i.e. the decrease in
peripheral resistance, unaffected. Can fluid cause a significant increase in cardiac output? A recent study[5] has shown that patients
given substantial volumes of Hartmann's solution, who did not become hypotensive, did have an increase in output but it was of a
minor order (10%) and it had disappeared by the time the patient

was ready for surgery. In spite of the fluid, 25% of the patients studied did develop hypotension and were given ephedrine.

Just how effective is pre-loading in preventing hypotension? Another recent paper,[6] reporting a study comparing electrolyte with colloid solutions, showed a large failure rate (40% with electrolyte and over 60% with colloid) in preventing hypotension. A review of the literature in the same paper showed very few studies in which reasonable prophylaxis against hypotension was achieved. Indeed, few studies had been undertaken with an adequate control group **not** given fluids.

If vasodilation is the primary cause of the decrease in arterial pressure, why are vasopressors not used as first line treatment? They are rapidly effective and have in any case to be given to a substantial number of mothers because the fluid failed to prevent hypotension.

The main fears are that vasoconstriction may adversely affect uterine blood flow,[6,7,8] and, following delivery, the augmented venous return may lead to severe hypertension if there is a substantial increase in peripheral resistance.

While pure α-adrenoreceptor stimulators such as methoxamine can reduce uterine blood flow,[7] the reverse is usually the case with combined α- and β-stimulators such as ephedrine.[9] The increase in uterine blood flow is of course secondary to the increase in arterial pressure and cardiac output.

The risk of severe hypertension at delivery is a problem if a large dose of a relatively long-acting agent has been used. However, this would not be the case if short-acting vasopressors (e.g. phenylephrine or noradrenaline) were given by infusion in sufficient amounts to maintain the systolic pressure around 100–120 mmHg. At delivery, the infusion can be stopped and any residual effects of the vasopressor will be short-lived. If ephedrine is used, and it is the most commonly used vasopressor for this purpose, it is best to use small bolus doses (5–10 mg) repeated as necessary. Sympathomimetics will also reverse all the other unpleasant effects of vagal overactivity such as nausea and vomiting. Atropine, often the first choice if bradycardia is present, is not very effective because while it opposes vagal stimulation if enough is given, it does not have any adrenergic effects.

In so far as prophylaxis is concerned, the most important measure is to avoid caval compression. Following injection of the main dose for epidural blockade, the patient should be kept fully lateral. There is still a belief that the spread of anaesthetic solutions in the epidural space is affected by gravity, though all the evidence is to the contrary, especially in the doses and volumes used for caesarean section. With spinal anaesthesia, gravity is of some importance and it is advisable to turn the patient from one side to the other 2 to 3 minutes after injecting the local anaesthetic.

When the patient is ready for surgery, use a wedge giving the maximum lateral tilt that the obstetrician will accept. Monitor the pulse and blood pressure frequently and treat bradycardia and/or hypotension with a vasopressor. Do not treat hypotension with fluid or atropine. The use of these agents will only lead to delay in restoring the blood pressure and heart rate.

While large volumes of intravenous fluid are not harmful to healthy parturients, they may be so to those with heart disease.[10] In any event, not doing harm is hardly a justification for an illogical, unsubstantiated and ineffective course of action.

* *

ARGUMENTS AGAINST: T. Bryson

Regional block in obstetrics frequently causes falls in blood pressure. In the main, this is due to vasodilation in the area of the block, as autonomic blockade inevitably accompanies sensory block. The extent of the autonomic blockade is always greater than the sensory block. This results in an enlargement of the vascular bed which gives rise to a relative hypovolaemia. In order to maintain the venous return to the heart, the flow-rate of blood through the circulatory system must increase and often this is sufficient to maintain the cardiac output. In obstetrics, however, the effects of aortocaval compressions by the uterus are always present to a greater or lesser degree and this often tips the balance into frank hypotension.[11]

The administration of a suitable quantity of intravenous fluid can compensate for the enlargement of the vascular bed[12,13] but of course additional methods are required to alleviate the aortocaval compression. It is better for the mother and fetus to prevent falls in blood pressure than to treat these when they have occurred. Fluid loading should therefore take place as the regional block develops rather than after vasodilation has occurred.

Pre-loading is a method of preventing hypotension due to vasodilation, which is the commonest complication of regional block in obstetrics and potentially the most dangerous to mother and fetus. The degree of hypotension is directly related to the extent of the block. The extensive blockade required for caesarean section will almost always require pre-loading but pre-loading is rarely required for analgesia in labour as the cause of hypotension then is usually caval compression. The practice of routinely pre-loading prior to 'top-ups' for normal labour is deprecated.

This discussion on pre-loading for regional blockade in obstetrics will refer only to the more extensive blockade required, for example, in caesarean section. The two techniques involved are epidural block and sub-arachnoid block. The main difference between these techniques is that the speed of onset of the block with spinals is accompanied by a more rapid development of vasodilation and hypotension.

Effects of hypotension on the mother

Hypotension in the mother during caesarean section under regional blockade gives rise to a feeling of faintness, sweating and general sensation of malaise. This makes the procedure an unpleasant experience for the mother and her attendants quite apart from the potential dangers of underperfusion of her tissues and vital organs, including the uterus and placenta. Significant hypotension will slow or stop the progress of labour. Maternal nausea and vomiting may make caesarean section more hazardous and difficult.

Hypotension will also affect the fetus, resulting at best in a stormy early postnatal life and at worst in possibly permanent effects on the fetal outcome.

Causes of hypotension during regional blockade

Vasodilation

This is caused by autonomic blockade resulting in a decrease of arterial tone and peripheral resistance and an increase in venous capacitance. There is resultant relative hypovolaemia and a decrease in venous return to the heart which results in a reduction of stroke volume and cardiac output. Blood pressure may be maintained at reasonable levels in the absence of caval compression.

Aortocaval compression

This is present in all cases if the mother is supine and sometimes also in other positions. The work of the Edinburgh group[14] clearly demonstrates that this will persist until the uterus is emptied. The contribution made by aortocaval compression will persist during the relatively short period from the mother being placed supine until the uterus is emptied.

Caval compression is now well recognised by obstetric anaesthetists so it is surprising that several misconceptions about it still exist. Two of the commonest are that if the blood pressure is within normal limits, no compression exists, and secondly that tilting the patient or displacing the uterus invariably relieves caval compression.

The effects of caval compression on the cardiac output and the blood pressure are seen only during the short period between the onset of autonomic blockade and the delivery of the fetus and the placenta. This is approximately 60–90 minutes for epidural block and

10–60 minutes for spinal block. Measures to prevent falls in blood pressure therefore need to be of relatively short duration.

Other factors

The decrease in arterial tone and the increase in venous capacity gives rise to a labile cardiovascular state in the mother. This may lead to dramatic blood pressure changes if the patient is moved frequently and carelessly under regional blockade, causing the circulatory volume to slop about in the enlarged vascular channels.[15]

Increased venous capacitance may also lead to pooling of blood in dependent limbs or the lower part of the body. Care must be taken to position the patient so that this does not occur.

The hypotension which occurs with regional block in obstetrics has two components. One is the vasodilation due to autonomic blockade and the second is due to aortocaval compression. Pre-loading will only deal with the effect of the former and in all cases steps have to be taken to prevent or minimise caval compression. To combat the effects of vasodilation, there are only two alternatives. Either the enlarged vascular space must be filled, which is most easily accomplished by pre-loading, or the peripheral resistance and venous capacitance must be restored to normal by the use of suitable vasopressors. The pre-loading solution is preferred for many reasons.

Pre-loading

Ease of treatment

A free-running intravenous infusion is required before starting a caesarean section or a regional block. It is easy therefore to administer a pre-load of up to two litres of a suitable intravenous fluid without further upset to the mother. This should take place before and during the development of autonomic blockade.

Safety of treatment

Pre-loading with up to two litres of intravenous (IV) fluid has been shown to be safe. Many fluid regimes have been advocated; for example, all crystalloid, all colloid, or mixtures of colloid and crystalloid. It is not my brief to enter into the crystalloid-versus-colloid controversy but this has recently been reviewed by Murray *et al.*[16] Crystalloids are effective and their use removes the rare possibility of anaphylactoid reaction to colloids. There is a possibility of overloading the circulation of the mother with the volume of fluid given. In healthy patients this does not occur. Wollman and Marx[12] using spinal anaesthesia, and Lewis *et al.*[13] using epidural analgesia found no evidence of fluid overloading either clinically or by measuring central venous pressure. Crystalloid solutions may be safer in this respect as they are more quickly eliminated from the body.

No harmful effects have been noted in the fetus from pre-loading as assessed by Apgar scores and fetal umbilical blood gas measurement.[12] Pre-loading has no effect on the maternal or neonatal blood glucose levels.[17] No significant changes are seen in coagulation indices or electrolyte levels, although the plasma colloid osmotic pressure may fall transiently.[18]

Crystalloid solutions do not remain in the intravascular compartment for long. Various estimates have been made and these have been calculated as being in the range of 20 minutes to two hours. Clinically, however, the effects in maintaining the circulating volume last at least two hours which adequately covers the period between the onset of the regional block and delivery of the fetus.

Bardgett (personal communication) studied the hourly urinary output following delivery in two groups of 20 elective caesarean sections. One group had general anaesthesia without pre-load and the second group had epidural analgesia with a two litre crystalloid pre-load. Both groups had a **diuresis** peak of 1.5 litres between ten and 16 hours after delivery but the epidural group had another peak of 1.5 litres in the first six hours following delivery. The first peak would appear to be the excretion of the pre-load which is therefore quickly excreted but is retained long enough to be effective. After delivery, the mother has to reduce the fluid retained during pregnancy to the normal non-pregnant state and the second peaks seen in both groups could be the beginning of this process. Wennberg *et al.*[18] confirm that most of the pre-load in their cases was excreted in the urine in the first three hours after delivery.

Efficacy of pre-loading

Pre-loading has been shown to be effective in preventing falls in blood pressure in both intrathecal and epidural anaesthesia. Wollman and Marx,[12] in a small series of mothers undergoing caesarean section under spinal analgesia, completely prevented falls in the systolic arterial pressure of more than 20% by pre-loading. This was in contrast to a control group who received no IV fluid pre-load. This group all had falls in blood pressure greater than 20%. The decrease in blood pressure was greatest in those mothers with the most extensive blocks. The falls in blood pressure were successfully treated by the infusion of IV fluid but both mother and fetus had been subjected to a period of hypotension which resulted in lowered Apgar scores and increased base deficits in the umbilical blood in the group which did not receive a pre-load. Lewis *et al.*[13] studied the effect of pre-loading on 60 mothers undergoing caesarean section with epidural analgesia to T4. Only four (6.7%) had a fall in systolic blood pressure greater than 20% and none had a fall exceeding 30%. No treatment for hypotension was required by any of the parturients.

Pre-loading therefore is successful in preventing hypotension in the majority of pregnant women with extensive regional block. The few failures of the method can be treated by further IV fluid or by small bolus doses of a vasopressor such as ephedrine. The initial pre-load must be of adequate volume and caval compression must be prevented by suitable measures. Using such a regime, vasopressors will rarely be required.

Disadvantages of pre-loading

The main objection to the use of pre-loading is that it involves giving further fluid to a woman who, due to her pregnancy, has already retained a considerable volume of additional fluid. It could be antici-pated that the extra fluid might cause pulmonary and circulatory embarrassment. There is no evidence that this occurs in a normal healthy woman but caution is obviously required if there is any evi-dence of cardiovascular or respiratory dysfunction or if the mother has pre-eclampsia. Clinical examination of pregnant women after pre-load has not revealed any evidence of pulmonary oedema.[12] Central venous pressure measurements following pre-load are increased but remain well below the levels seen in pulmonary oedema. It has been suggested that observation of neck vein filling is the only monitoring require-ment.[13]

It might be anticipated that electrolyte, haemoglobin and glucose levels would be altered by dilution but this does not occur.[17,18]

Urethral catheterisation is required in patients receiving IV pre-load for caesarean section under regional blockade. This is necessary to prevent the bladder intruding into the operative field. Some would regard this as a disadvantage, but as it has become almost a routine practice in obstetrics, it may be regarded as a relatively minor one.

Use of vasopressors

The only practical alternative way of treating hypotension following regional blockade is by the administration of vasopressor drugs. If this is done, caval compression must be prevented by the usual methods. Vasopressors will not restore the blood pressure in the presence of aortocaval compression.[19]

The duration of any maternal hypotension is important, as in-creased duration of hypotension increases the likelihood of neonatal depression with both spinal and epidural analgesia.[12,20] Prevention of hypotension is more advantageous to the fetus and the mother than prompt treatment of established hypotension. The prophylactic use of vasopressors is disappointing and has a high incidence of failure.[20,21] These drugs therefore are mainly used to combat falls in blood pressure which are already present and may be causing symptoms.

The administration of any drug to the mother may result in significant blood levels and pharmacological effects in the fetus. Vasopressors are no exception to this process. Although there is evidence that the placenta breaks down some of these drugs, placental transfer still occurs.[22] Vasopressors are drugs with a wide range of actions. As well as acting directly on the heart and the peripheral circulation, they also have effects on the bronchi, pupils, gastro-intestinal tract, central nervous system and the uterus. In the uterus, there is a reduction in uterine activity and changes in uterine blood flow have been seen. The uterine blood flow is reduced, particularly if hypertension occurs following the administration of the drugs.[22] Ralston *et al.* have shown in animal models that this latter effect is most marked with methoxamine and metaraminol.

The drug most favoured by obstetric anaesthetists at the present time is ephedrine. Part of its peripheral action is due to noradrenaline release. It has a relatively long duration of action but tachyphylaxis is seen and rapidly repeated doses give less effective responses.[23]

Ephedrine

Ephedrine is an old remedy, having been used in China for about 2000 years, and was introduced into Western medicine in 1924. It is undoubtedly an effective and useful drug but is even more an 'old wives' tale' than the more recently introduced technique of preloading. It stimulates both α and β receptors and has a long duration of action. It has pronounced central actions. The cardiovascular effects are similar to those of adrenaline but persist about ten times as long. The pressor effects are partly due to vasoconstriction but the main effect is by cardiac stimulation. The force of myocardial contraction is increased, as is the cardiac output. Uterine activity is decreased and it has similar central effects to amphetamine. Ephedrine is excreted in breast milk and irritability and disturbed sleep have been reported in breastfed infants.

In general, therefore, ephedrine has a widespread action on the body and although it is undoubtedly effective in raising blood pressure, its use could be compared to using a machine gun on a single target when a sniper's rifle might be more effective and less dangerous to the surrounding onlookers.

Robson *et al.*[5] studied the changes in cardiac output in a group of 20 healthy women during epidural anaesthesia for caesarean section using a non-invasive technique of Doppler ultrasound and echocardio-graphic measurement. The cardiac output was measured before starting the epidural, after crystalloid pre-loading and at ten-minute intervals thereafter until the start of surgery. The blood pressure was measured at one-minute intervals and if it fell by more than 20% from the base level, the rate of the IV infusion was increased and a 5–10 mg IV bolus dose of ephedrine was given. Only five of the mothers had a fall in blood pressure greater than 20%. The cardiac output rose following the pre-load in all cases, but fell to the basal level before surgery started. In the five women who were given eph-edrine, two (40%) had a hypertensive response (MAP >100 mmHg) and more importantly, three (60%) had a gross increase in cardiac output, exceeding ten litres per minute in all three cases. The authors stressed, in view of this, the need for caution in the administration of ephedrine. They also confirmed the beneficial effects of crystalloid pre-load on the venous return and cardiac stroke volume.

The use of ephedrine is not without hazard to mother and fetus, although its occasional use may be of great value in severe cases of hypotension. The most important concept in regional block in obstet-rics is the **prevention** of hypotension. This is best achieved by a combination of measures to prevent aortocaval compression and IV fluid pre-loading. This is recognised by most practising obstetric anaesthetists who have adopted fluid pre-loading as an essential part of their anaesthetic technique, thus minimising their incidence of hypotension. The degree of success may be improved by other measures such as compression bandaging of the lower limbs.[24]

Vasopressors have a small part to play in the treatment of those cases which are refractory to pre-loading.

It is right to question slavish acceptance of the technique, as has been done recently,[25] as this allows us to re-examine pre-loading and its effects and also to assess any alternatives. This I have tried to do in this presentation. At the present time, there is no suitable alternative to pre-loading which is a safe, well-tolerated, effective method in-volving little risk to the mother and the fetus. Perhaps at some future time, we may be given a 'pure' vasopressor drug acting only on the peripheral vessels with a short duration of action, effective as a prophylactic and which will not cause rebound hypertension. Then perhaps we could re-run this debate but until then, fluid pre-loading is the best and safest method of preventing hypotension in regional blockade in obstetrics.

REFERENCES

1. Kerr MG, Scott DB, Samuel E. Studies of the inferior vena cava in late pregnancy. *British Medical Journal* 1964; **1:** 532–3.
2. Lees MM, Kerr MG, Scott DB, Taylor SH. Circulatory effects of the supine posture in late pregnancy. *Clinical Science* 1967; **32:** 453–65.
3. Bieniarz J, Maqueda R, Caldeyro-Barcia R. Compression of the aorta by the uterus in late human pregnancy: I. Variations between femoral and brachial artery pressure with changes from hypertension to hypotension. *American Journal of Obstetrics and Gynecology* 1966; **95:** 795–808.
4. Bonica JJ, Berges PU, Morikawa K. Circulatory effects of peridural block: I. Effects of levels of analgesia and dose of lidocaine. *Anesthesiology* 1970; **33:** 619–26.
5. Robson S, Hunter S, Boys R, Dunlop W, Bryson M. Changes in cardiac output during epidural anaesthesia for Caesarean section. *Anaesthesia* 1989; **44:** 475–9.
6. Shnider SM, de Lorimier AA, Hall JW, Chapler FK, Morishima HO. Vasopressors in obstetrics. I. Correction of fetal acidosis with ephedrine during spinal hypotension. *American Journal of Obstetrics and Gynecology* 1968; **102:** 911–19.
7. Shnider SM, de Lorimier AA, Hall JW. Vasopressors in obstetrics. II. Fetal hazards of methoxamine administration during obstetric spinal anaesthesia. *American Journal of Obstetrics and Gynecology* 1970; **106:** 680–6.
8. Shnider SM, de Lorimier AA, Steenson JL. Vasopressors in obstetrics. III. Fetal effects of metaraminol infusion during obstetric spinal hypotension. *American Journal of Obstetrics and Gynecology* 1970; **108:** 1017–22.
9. Hollmen AI, Jouppila R, Albright GA, Jouppila P, Vierola H, Koivula A. Intervillous blood flow during Caesarean section with prophylactic ephedrine and epidural anaesthesia. *Acta Anaesthesiol Scand* 1984; **28:** 396–400.
10. Alderson JD. Cardiovascular collapse following epidural anaesthesia for Caesarean section in a patient with aortic incompetence. *Anaesthesia* 1987; **42:** 643–5.
11. Scott DB. Inferior vena caval occlusion during epidural block. In: Doughty A, ed. *Proceedings of the symposium on epidural analgesia in obstetrics.* London: HK Lewis, 1972.
12. Wollman SB, Marx GF. Acute hydration for prevention of hypotension of spinal anesthesia in parturients. *Anesthesiology* 1968; **29:** 374–80.
13. Lewis M, Thomas P, Wilkes RG. Hypotension during epidural analgesia for Caesarean section. *Anaesthesia* 1983; **38:** 250–3.
14. Scott DB. Inferior vena caval occlusion in late pregnancy and its importance in anaesthesia. *British Journal of Anaesthesia* 1968; **40:** 120–8.
15. Thorburn J. Factors modifying epidural block for Caesarean section. In: Reynolds F, ed. *Epidural and spinal blockade in obstetrics.* London: Bailliere Tindall, 1990.
16. Murray AM, Morgan M, Whitwam JG. Crystalloid versus colloid for circulatory preload for epidural Caesarean section. *Anaesthesia* 1989; **44:** 463–6.

17. Thomas P, Buckley P, Fox M. Maternal and neonatal blood glucose after crystalloid loading for epidural Caesarean section. *Anaesthesia* 1983; **83:** 250–3.
18. Wennberg E, Frid I, Haljamae M, Kjellner I. Comparison of Ringer's acetate with 3% Dextran for volume loading before extradural Caesarean section. *British Journal of Anaesthesia* 1990; **65:** 654–60.
19. Marx GF, Bassell GM. Hazards of the supine position in pregnancy. In: Rosen M, ed. *Obstetric anaesthesia and analgesia: safer practice.* London: WB Saunders, 1982.
20. Rolbin SH, Cole AFD, Hew EM, Pollard A, Virgint S. Prophylactic IM ephedrine before epidural anaesthesia for Caesarean section: efficacy and actions on the foetus and newborn. *Canadian Anaesthetists Society Journal* 1982; **29:** 148–53.
21. Moya F, Smith BE. Spinal anaesthesia for Caesarean section. *Journal of the American Medical Association* 1962; **179:** 609.
22. Ralston DH, Shnider SM, de Lorimier AA. Effects of equipotent ephedrine metaraminal mephentermine and methoxamine on uterine blood flow in the pregnant ewe. *Anesthesiology* 1974; **40:** 354–69.
23. Goodman LS, Gilman AG. *The pharmacological basis of therapeutics.* Gilman AG, Rall TW, Nies AS, Taylor P. (eds) 8th edition. New York and Oxford: Pergamon Press, 1990.
24. Bhagwanjee S, Rocke DA, Rout CC, Koovarjee RV, Brijball R. Prevention of hypotension following spinal anaesthesia for elective Caesarean section by wrapping of the legs. *British Journal of Anaesthesia* 1990; **65:** 819–22.
25. Editorial. Epidural block for Caesarean section and circulatory changes. *Lancet* 1989; **ii:** 1076–8.

3

Anaesthetists exaggerate their role by demanding the closure of smaller obstetric units.

ARGUMENTS FOR: W. Savage

I have always very much appreciated the help that I have had from my anaesthetic colleagues, and think that they are an absolutely essential part of the team. However, I do think that they have exaggerated their role in respect of small obstetric units, as described in the booklet *Anaesthetic Services for Obstetrics—A Plan for the Future*.[1] This well-produced pamphlet had extremely wide circulation—it was circulated to all District Health Authorities (DHAs), with wide recommendations made by the group of anaesthetists who did the work. My criticism of this document is that it is very much like the White Paper *Working for Patients*, very strong on statements of what should be done without being backed up by sufficiently wide-ranging, good documentary evidence.

Maternal mortality
As most of the audience are anaesthetists, I will just remind you of what has happened to maternal mortality over the last 100 years (Fig. 3.1).[2] You can see that for about 100 years there was a rate of four deaths per 1000 women in association with childbirth. The rate began to fall in the mid-1930s, and that was because of a decline in puerperal sepsis associated with a decrease in the virulence of the streptococcus and helped by the manufacture of the first sulphonamide. It fell most rapidly in the 1940s and 1950s, when most of the obstetricians and the anaesthetists were away fighting the war, and most of the women were able to get on with birth with the help of midwives(!), the NHS was created, penicillin and streptomycin became available, and blood transfusion services were set up. Over the last 20 years, there has been a more modest decline, although plotted on a log scale one can

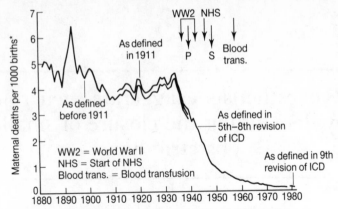

Fig. 3.1 Trends in maternal mortality, England and Wales, 1881–1981 (from Macfarlane A, Mugford M. *Birth counts*. London: HMSO, 1984)

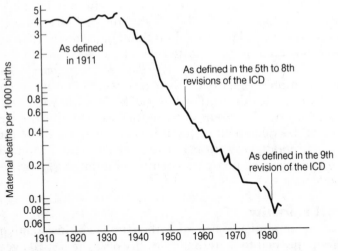

Source: OP-CS mortality statistics

Fig. 3.2 Maternal mortality, England and Wales, 1911–84, plotted on a logarithmic scale (from *Confidential enquiries into maternal deaths in England and Wales, 1982–84*)

see that the rate of death has halved each decade since 1930 (Fig. 3.2). In addition, over the past 20 years anaesthesia has edged its way up, becoming one of the leading causes of maternal mortality (Table 3.1).

Perinatal mortality

If we look at perinatal mortality (and in honour of my Chairman, I have put up the rates for Scotland, 64/1000 in 1940 and 12/1000 in 1985), you can see that for the last 50 years the majority of women

Table 3.1   Cause of death. Rates per million maternities E and W from 1964–66. Rank order in brackets

Cause of death	61–63	64–66	67–69	70–72	73–75	76–78	79–81	82–84
Hypertensive diseases	41.3 (3)	25.8 (4)	21.6 (3)	20.5 14.9 (3)	20.3 13.2 (1)	16.6 12.5 (2)	14.2 (1)	10.0 (1)
Pulmonary embolism	51.2 (2)	35.0 (2)	30.5 (2)	26.5 17.6 (2)	18.2 12.8 (2)	25.7 18.5 (1)	9.0 (2)	10.0 (1)
Abortion	55.1 (1)	51.1 (1)	47.6 (1)	35.2 25.3 (1)	15.1 10.5 (3)	10.9 6.0 (5)	5.5 (6)	4.4 (5)
Haemorrhage	36.5 (4)	26.2 (3)	16.7 (5)	11.7 10.4 (5)	10.9 8.1 (5)	14.9 10.3 (4)	5.5 (6)	3.6 (7)
Anaesthesia	na	19.2 (6)	20.3 (4)	12.8 (4)	10.5 (3)	11.6 (3)	8.7 (3)	7.2 (3)

From Tables 19.4 and 19.5 in *Report on Confidential Enquiries into Maternal Deaths in England and Wales 1982–4*. The differences in rates follow a classification change in ICD9. Anaesthetic deaths were not calculated separately until 1970–2 Report, so figures for the two earlier reports were calculated in retrospect.

have given birth to live and healthy babies. All our effort over the past 45 years has decreased the rate only a little.[3]

An increasing proportion of women, midwives and some obstetricians are beginning to question whether the way that we have organised the maternity services is actually the right way to do it. Hospital birth, increasing interference with the natural process of birth, increasing use of powerful drugs or techniques to control the pain of labour have led to a 25% rate of caesarean section in the richest country in the world. In the UK the rate is probably approaching 12%, i.e., 120 women per 1000, double the fall in PMR since 1930.[4,5] The fall in PMR from 33 in 1958 to 11 in 1985 was accompanied by a rise in the CS rate from 2.8 to 10%, i.e. 70 women per 1000 having operations and 20 less babies per 1000 dying in association with childbirth mainly because of increasingly successful care of the preterm infant.

Marjorie Tew (a statistician), in the course of teaching medical students in the 1970s, came across a rather strange anomaly in the birth statistics; that as home birth declined, the perinatal mortality did not fall as fast as it ought to have done if it was safer to have your baby in hospital.[6] She has this to say about obstetricians.

The majority of obstetricians everywhere have become convinced that the natural process of birth is fraught with dangers that their increasingly sophisticated interventions are increasingly capable of minimising. Amazingly, they have managed, without producing any supporting evidence, to convince the majority of people, both medical and lay, that they are right, and the maternity service has been organised in accordance with this unjustifiable hypothesis.[7]

Strong words, you might say, and related to the fact that it has taken Marjorie over 10 years to get her work accepted. So it was particularly disappointing to find that the anaesthetists were jumping in on the act just as we were beginning to gather some support for the idea that perhaps there might be some benefit for women in either having their babies at home or in small units. When Roma Campbell and Alison MacFarlane—again statisticians, not obstetricians—reviewed the evidence in 1987, they concluded that:

> There is no evidence to support the claim that the shift to hospital deliveries is responsible for the decline in perinatal mortality in England and Wales, nor the claim that the safest policy is for all women to be delivered in hospital.[8]

The policy of centralising births in one large regional unit is quite disastrous in places like Scotland, where women may have to travel 80 miles to hospital, only to give birth in the ambulance. What anxiety does this cause the woman? Am I in labour/am I not in labour? Should I call the ambulance now/should I not? What happens when there is snow on the road? What does this anxiety do to the process of labour? What does it do to the woman?

How safe is birth in small units?
When we go back to maternal mortality, we can see that the proportion of deaths due to anaesthesia has not declined as fast as deaths due to other causes in obstetrics. I have taken the figures from the individual triennial inquiries, to document the causes of death. Some of these deaths are associated with spontaneous or induced abortion, some with ectopic pregnancy and some with sterilisation following delivery. None of those things would you expect to find going on in a small GP unit or probably even a small obstetric unit, isolated from the main hospital.

From 1970–76 there were four deaths associated with manual removal of placenta, which is of course one of the things that may be carried out in a small obstetric unit, even if it is not doing caesarean sections. However, the last time that GP obstetricians were mentioned was in the 1970–72 report and since then they have not been mentioned as being responsible for any maternal deaths. So GP obstetric units giving anaesthetics for manual removals appear to be safe.

What is the cause of anaesthetic deaths?

The proportion of avoidable factors in anaesthetic deaths has risen from 75.7% in 1970–72 to 95% in 1976–78. The number of deaths due to epidural, avoidable because there were errors of technique, has risen as the number of epidurals has risen, and when you read what the authors of the confidential inquiries have to say about these deaths, I think it is really debatable whether closing small units is going to make any difference. Since 22 of the deaths with avoidable factors involved junior staff, better supervision or use of more experienced doctors would be expected to reduce the number of deaths. In the 1973–75 and 1976–78 reports there are some really trenchant comments:

> In this report there are examples of SHOs who exercised knowledge and skill in adverse circumstances, whilst others acted from no discernible knowledge of the basis of anaesthesia in general or obstetric anaesthesia in particular . . . These deaths are attributable to a combination of lack of knowledge, inexperience, low general standards of care in labour.[9–13]

Now what has this got to do with small units who may be staffed by experienced, older GPs and anaesthetists? It is to do with how we train and supervise our junior staff, and I think that is where the effort needs to be put.

Where is the evidence?

In this report of the working party,[1] consultation did take place with two paediatricians and one senior obstetrician. As you all know, if you have four obstetricians in a room, you will probably have five views on how to manage a problem (and if you ask them the same questions six months later using the same data, their own opinions will differ from those decisions made earlier). So if you want an obstetric opinion to confirm your viewpoint, it is quite easy to get someone from the conservative/interventionist end of the spectrum. But what is notable is that they did not, apparently, consult one midwife, one GP or any women. Now, they make allowance for this by saying that there were five women out of the 12 on this committee (and that is pretty amazing coming from obstetrics, where we don't have one committee with anything like that number of women on it), but the report itself does, I think, overstate the case and appears to put forward the idea that women **need** ('approximately one third of mothers require . . .') an anaesthetist during childbirth. Well, how do they arrive at that figure? They don't give you any evidence for that in terms of asking women. It is true that in 1985, the last year for which we have statistics, 10.5% of women had a caesarean section, so we would have needed an anaesthetist for that. About 3.5% had a rotational forceps, so that is 14% of women requiring anaesthesia. Approximately 17% of women had an epidural, but there is some overlap with the operative delivery group and if you say that a third to a half of the epidurals were not associated with complicated births, you are getting up to 20–23%.

Does a woman really **require** an epidural for normal labour? A small percentage of women do have very painful labours, and find it hard to cope with, but currently at the London Hospital, only 5% of women have an epidural and that is because we do not have an epidural service. I am not sure that that is a bad thing because once you do have an epidural service, you have got the situation where there is an anaesthetist prowling round the labour ward looking for work. Of course he finds it, and if the way that childbirth is presented to women in the antenatal classes makes it seem that the pain is so terrible that you can't go through labour without an epidural, women may well request it.

Every time there is a death or a brain-damaged woman following an epidural, the rate of epidural requests goes down within all those hospitals within reading distance, and I think that we are poor at fully informing women about the disadvantages of epidural anaesthesia. If they were fully informed (p6, 'potentially life-threatening complications may occur at any time during an epidural block')[1] I doubt very much whether they would be wanting to have one for the average labour. It is fascinating that on page 3, the booklet says about anaesthesia in obstetrics, 'In recent years, women have become increasingly aware of the benefits of adequate analgesia during labour and delivery. Many mothers now expect this service to be provided routinely. (there is no reference for that statement). The anaesthetist provides expertise in all aspects of analgesia for the obstetric patient, including the use of narcotics, inhalational agents and regional techniques.' Well that may be true, but where is the evidence for that? In our underfunded, inner city region, they certainly have not had time to advise us about the use of narcotics, or inhalational agents for that matter. (Since I gave this lecture we now have an anaesthetist with a responsibility for obstetric anaesthesia.)

Where evidence is cited it is not always right
'The value of relieving maternal distress and reducing perinatal morbidity has been clearly shown—ref 9' (p3).[1]

I looked up reference 9 because I recognised the authors, and it is an article in the BMJ about social support in labour. This randomised study showed that women who were supported by a female companion had a caesarean section rate which was half that of those who had no such support. Their need for analgesia (which, in this Guatamalan study, was pretty low) and their need for syntocinon to augment labour was reduced. Placing this reference in a paragraph about women's desire for routine analgesic services seems bizarre.[14]

Some of us would think that perhaps the way to reduce the number of anaesthetic deaths would be to have a little less anaesthesia. If you did not have any epidurals, you would not have any deaths from epidural analgesia. If you did fewer operative deliveries there would be less need for anaesthesia; GP units and women booked for home birth in the UK as well as Holland have a very low rate of operative vaginal delivery.[2,15]

I just want to show you the results of a GP unit, in which a contemporary of mine gives anaesthetics. At one of the Old Londoners meetings, he was talking to me about this and he said, 'Well, I suppose I will have to give up giving anaesthetics. I have been doing it for 25 years and have never had any problems, but the anaesthetists at the hospital are saying that it is not safe'. Why is he not safe, compared to some of these SHOs, or even some young consultants? He has been doing it for 25 years, he knows what it is about, he is careful, he has got a simple technique in which he is an expert. In Table 3.2 you see that among the 597 women that were delivered in 1987, there was a very low perinatal mortality rate. There were six cases of retained placentae, no twins, two undiagnosed breeches transferred early, and 20 forceps deliveries, but they were not rotational forceps, so did not need anaesthesia. So you can select women carefully for these units, and you can provide a safe service.

Table 3.2   GP Unit

889 ♀ Booked
198 → Consultant care antenatally
87 → Consultant Unit in labour
(20 in premature labour, i.e. <8% transfer term)
597 ♀ Delivered
PNMR 2.9 (258 1<36/52 1>36/52)
GPs give anaesthetics if needed
6 Retained placentae
0 Twins
2 Undiagnosed breech transferred early
20 Forceps (no Caesars in GPU)

GP units without an anaesthetic service

When it was put to Professor Rosen that if you don't have an anaesthetic service, it can't be substandard, he said 'Oh well, I didn't mean my report to apply to units which don't give anaesthetics'. Unfortunately that is not how it reads, and that certainly is not how it is read by planners and district general managers, desperate to save some money to keep the show on the road.

Gavin Young, a GP obstetrician, did a survey of GP units in 1988, and he got a 55% response rate to one mailing. He found that of the 55 units that were still GP units without the facility to do caesarean sections, 29 were able to provide general anaesthetics (GA) and 20 did so during the year. Twenty would not give GA, none provided an epidural service. Of the 9000 women who gave birth in these units, 41 had a GA. So, nationally there would probably be less than 100 GAs given by GPs. In country areas, GPs are still giving anaesthetics (Table 3.3).

Table 3.3   Gavin Young Survey 1988

119 GP units E & W	
65 Responded (55%)	3 closed
	2 integrated
	2 IP Care
58	
3 did CS and had anaesthetist	
55 Units	29 could give GA (20 did)
	26 would not give GA
None gave epidurals	
9237 ♀	41 GA
Estimate < 100 GA's given by GPs mostly for MRP	

When I was in New Zealand, I worked in a hospital with over 400 beds, several surgeons of various types, three obstetricians and gynaecologists, and two anaesthetists. Both of these men were in their late fifties and they could not possibly do all the emergency anaesthesia, so when the House Officers came, they had a two week course in how to give a safe anaesthetic. In the three years that I was there, we never had a problem with the House Officers giving an unsafe anaesthetic. So why GPs who have learned how to give anaesthetics should forget how to give them, I do not know. Are they more or less likely to connect the anaesthetic machine badly (a reason for at least three deaths in one of those confidential inquiries). They know their apparatus, they know how to use it, they know they have not had to do it for quite some time, and they are probably more careful.

Natural birth is possible for most women and enjoyable for some. There is also some evidence that low-tech childbirth is safer than high-tech childbirth, and some of that evidence comes from a study done in New Zealand by Rosenblatt et al.[16] They found that the perinatal mortality was lower in the small hospitals doing less than 1000 deliveries per year than it was in the big hospitals. Another example comes from The Farm in Tennessee (a hippie commune which started in the 1970s) where self-trained midwives had achieved a good PMR with a CS rate of 1.5% in 1600 births from 1972–88.[17]

How did they do it? They did it by continuity of care, by personal care and a quiet, relaxed, home birth situation. This is the antithesis of the central, huge hospital units, with 5000 women delivering, knowing none of the people, having shifts of doctors, shorter shifts of midwives and streams of people coming through the labour ward. It is not the right way to give birth. Birth, like sex, is a private activity, that few people like to perform in a group of virtual strangers.

Anxiety

I think that we need to reduce the need for anaesthesia by retaining these small units, and we need to select the high-risk women for hospital. With all our technology we seem to be even less confident in the UK at doing this now than we were 30 years ago when we were without it. I think it is because we have made ourselves far too anxious and now the anaesthetists are adding to that anxiety. Anaesthetists, like obstetricians, are only called in when there is something wrong. The majority of women are looked after by midwives and a few by GPs, and we should leave them to get on with it.

We also, I think, need to consider what is required for safe anaesthesia. The important thing is to have somebody who knows how to give an anaesthetic, and knows what to do when it goes wrong, and that is something you can learn and retain.

When I was in my small hospital in New Zealand, which did 1000 deliveries a year (and what would women do if they closed it because it would be miles and miles for the women to go, they would have to fly to Napier 150 miles away), I was doing a caesarean section one day, and the anaesthetist said to me, 'Can you do a tracheostomy?' I thought, 'Christ, a tracheostomy' and I remembered my lecture on tracheostomy and I remembered the one I had done eight years before, and I did an emergency tracheostomy. He could not intubate this young woman, and we got on and did the caesar, and she survived and so did the baby. But the thing is that one needs to have that kind of drill there in the theatre, and again, there in the last confidential inquiry, it is said that there should be a drill agreed by anaesthetists and obstetricans for the management of these anaesthetic problems, especially including haemorrhage.

I just want to read to you from a Dr Fairleigh, whom I have never met, who is a consultant obstetrician and gynaecologist in Forthpark Hospital, Kirkcaldy, Fife. He says, talking about Grantley Dick Read, that, 'He believed, with good antenatal care and education embracing the total phenomena of labour, that fear, tension, pain and unnecessary anaesthesia could be eliminated.' Most patients properly prepared for labour did not want anaesthesia. For most of his life Dr Dick Read was a prophet crying in the wilderness as far as the British medical profession was concerned, although by the end of his life, he saw his view welcomed by women across the world.

Most consultant obstetricians in the UK are nominally responsible for several hundred births per year, and have a heavy gynaecological commitment. The result is that much of the obstetric care is given by the disproportionately large number of doctors still in training. This lack of continuity is an important cause of apprehension, tension and pain in labour, and is most likely in large obstetric units. The report *Anaesthetic Services for Obstetrics—A Plan for the Future*, published by the Association of Anaesthetists and leaning heavily on a survey by the National Birthday Trust,[18] advises that maternity units in the UK should be reduced to match the number of skilled anaesthetists. Dr Dick Read had a suitable comment when many years ago, in *Childbirth Without Fear*, he wrote, 'When I read through the list of the services for the National Birthday Fund, I wish sincerely that one of them might have been the prevention of painful labour'. Let there be no mistaking his meaning; midwives, GPs and obstetricians can prevent painful labour . . .

In both epidural and general anaesthesia during labour, potentially life-threatening complications may occur and it would therefore be reasonable to explore the extent to which the obstetrician can safely reduce demands on the anaesthetist. In this respect, a revival in the technique of caesarean section under local anaesthetic would be in the interests of both mother and baby. Small maternity hospitals may make a greater contribution to childbirth safety than larger units, so I would say to you all, let us please be flexible in our way of looking at anaesthesia and accept with all due humility that perhaps some of the GPs and midwives working in these small hospitals know more about childbirth than we, who are the experts in the abnormal.'

Women know how and where they want to give birth and some will choose to go to a unit which provides a full range of services. Those who choose to have their baby at home or in a small friendly unit should be able to make that choice as long as they are healthy and the pregnancy has progressed normally. Experts in the abnormal should accept that their role, whilst important, is limited and leave decisions about the place of birth to those who know about normal birth; women, midwives and GPs.

*   *

ARGUMENTS AGAINST: B. Morgan

The reason anaesthetists must demand the closure of smaller units is because there are too many units for the existing anaesthetic man-power to service.[1] It is as simple as that.

The confidential enquiry into facilities available at place of birth has revealed the following details.[18] The little unit delivering less than

500 babies a year frequently has no anaesthetic service and the mother has no more access to anaesthetic facilities than she would have if she was having her baby at home—the ultimate small unit. These mothers are usually carefully selected as being at low risk and have chosen to be in a unit without anaesthesia. This is not only perfectly acceptable to anaesthetists but has nothing to do with them. So mothers, midwives and obstetricians need not be appalled at the closure of the dear, friendly little unit round the corner; this is not what the anaesthetists are aiming for. Closure of these units is simply on the grounds of economy, as these units are not viable in the present type of health service funding. These units cannot be closed on the grounds of substandard anaesthetic service as they do not have any anaesthetic service at all.

There are 217 very small units and these deliver about 1% of the children in the country; another 1% are delivered at home. Obviously we cannot staff these units any more than we could the hundreds of homes where births occur. Most of these units are staffed by GP obstetricians and, where anaesthetics are offered, these are usually done by GP anaesthetists.

It is the other 98% of women with whom we concern ourselves. They go to the 303 units with delivery rates above 500. Almost half of these units have less than 2000 deliveries a year and 30% of the children are born in them. The other half of the units with over 2000 deliveries a year have 70% of the births.[18]

The 149 units with fewer than 2000 deliveries per year do not take low-risk mothers as evidenced by the method of delivery and the need for anaesthesia. Their rate of caesarean sections, etc. is exactly the same as it is in the big units. But the provision of anaesthetic facilities is vastly different, with many having no anaesthetist on the premises and very few with an immediately available anaesthetist, some with no known consultant available, almost a third with the only anaesthetist being a junior. Most of these less than 2000 units attempt to offer an epidural service but it is often only occasional.

Of course, not all these smaller units are badly staffed; some have excellent, devoted consultants who live round the corner and offer a superb consultant-based service. But not many. Nor are all large units well staffed or provided with adequate facilities, as shown by this survey.[18] But it is these 149 units that take all comers at all times in which the obstetric fraternity with the aid of the anaesthetists seek to deceive and defraud mothers into thinking that they have some measure of safety in spite of having an obviously deficient anaesthetic service.

It is not surprising that many people question the increased safety of hospital deliveries when one examines the anaesthetic care of these smaller units. It is these units that must be closed or amalgamated or moved because the unselected mothers are at risk from a substandard level of anaesthetic care.

Whether all these 149 units are necessary or not, we do not have the anaesthetic manpower to staff them. Many of these 149 units strike me as being the obstetricians' ego trip. They don't want to give up their obstetric beds and to hell with the service mothers get. Neither obstetricians nor mothers can be expected to understand or uphold anaesthetic standards; that is what the consultant anaesthetist must do. Anaesthetists understand how unsafe it is. Being unable to staff all these units, we are party to the fact that the often ridiculously young anaesthetist is expected to rush, sometimes several miles, to a unit to give an instant anaesthetic in a hurry to a woman whom he has never seen before, frequently with poor facilities and often no assistance. It is not surprising that we manage to kill about ten women a year.

Most anaesthetists in this room are valiantly battling with the health authorities for improvements in their standards and it is right that national bodies, such as the Association of Anaesthetists and the RCOG, should help by setting standards. These standards attempt to ensure that the obstetric patient who needs anaesthesia receives the care that would be regarded as commonplace for the surgical patient.

Placental animals are endangered by maternal haemorrhage and fetal hypoxia at every delivery. These twin horrors both need an anaesthetist and an obstetrician. No obstetrician would willingly treat a mother with torrential haemorrhage alone, giving, as we did two weeks ago, 28 units of blood while opening the abdomen. Without immediate and trained anaesthetic help, such mothers would die and about four per year do just that. But the dangers of fetal hypoxia are so well known that a large part of obstetric work is fetal monitoring, especially during labour.

One may indeed question the purpose of such monitoring if no immediate action can be taken to deliver the child showing signs of hypoxia because you have to wait for the anaesthetist. Hypoxia wrecks the child's cerebral machinery at times too quickly to await the arrival of an anaesthetist for a caesarean section from a neighbouring hospital when at last freed from his surgical list or intensive care duties. We cannot but accept that as anaesthetists we have a vital role to play in reducing neonatal morbidity and mortality.

The reason why anaesthetists demand closure of some of these 149 units is clear; the substandard level of anaesthetic care that unselected mothers are offered unbeknown to them is indefensible. Withdrawal of anaesthetic service will not do; high-risk mothers will still be admitted and have to be treated. It is difficult and at times impossible to inform mothers that the care is substandard. The existence of this excessive number of units jeopardises the other units.

What about all the talk of hundreds of babies being delivered on the hard shoulder of the M4? For the most part, this is a densely populated little island with excellent communications. This is not Norway or Canada with geographical and climatic difficulties. What about the Highlands and the Shetlands, shrill voices yell. Well, of course, special provision needs to be made for these inaccessible places but no one chooses to live in these places for their excellent facilities, and because the provision of anaesthetic care might be poor in the Hebrides, it doesn't mean it has to be so in London. Within a radius of five miles of Queen Charlotte's Hospital there are eight obstetric units, most of which have small numbers. The aim should be one unit per district whenever possible.

It is not for obstetricians, Mrs Savage or any others to tell anaesthetists what standards of anaesthetic care they should provide or whether GP anaesthetists are safe. Obstetricians are as ignorant of anaesthetic requirements as anaesthetists are unable to lay down standards of obstetric practice.

The standard of anaesthetic care we must aim for is the provision of an anaesthetic service for mothers as good as that which would be regarded as commonplace for the surgical patient.

The anaesthetist responsible for obstetric anaesthesia, who is often based in a nearby hospital and who knows the facilities to be inadequate to allow immediate safe anaesthesia if necessary, is in my view guilty of irresponsible behaviour that should not be tolerated in a caring society and certainly not defended by obstetricians.

Clearly the people who have nothing to lose are those working in these units who fight to keep them open. Neither they nor the mothers who have already delivered their infants have anything at stake. The people with most to lose are the defenceless children who are most at risk of hypoxia, that might be mitigated by anaesthesia for an essential operative delivery.

I put it to you—which anaesthetist in this audience would be willing to have their own children born in such units? If we know they are unsafe, how can we continue to allow others to use them?

REFERENCES

1. Working Party of the Association of Anaesthetists of Great Britain and Ireland and the Obstetric Anaesthetists Association. *Anaesthetic services for obstetrics—A plan for the future*. London: 1987.
2. Macfarlane A, Mugford M. *Birth counts: statistics of pregnancy and childbirth*. London: HMSO, 1984.
3. Savage W. *A savage enquiry: who controls childbirth?* London: Virago, 1986.
4. Boyd C, Francomb C. *One birth in nine: caesarean section trends since 1978*. London: Maternity Alliance, 1983.

5.   Office of Population Censuses and Surveys. *Birth statistics 1837–1983.* London: HMSO, 1987.
6.   Tew M. Understanding intranatal care through mortality statistics. In: Zander L, Chamberlain G, eds. *Pregnancy care for the 1980s.* London: RSM/Macmillan Press.
7.   Tew M. Do obstetric interventions make birth safer? *British Journal of Gynaecology* 1986; **93:** 659–74.
8.   Campbell R, Macfarlane A. Place of delivery: a review. *British Journal of Gynaecology* 1986; **93:** 675–83.
9.   *Report of confidential enquiries into maternal deaths in England and Wales. Report on health and social subjects no. 11 1970–2.* London: HMSO, 1975.
10.   *Report on confidential enquiries into maternal deaths in England and Wales. Report on health and social subjects no. 14 1973–5.* London: HMSO, 1979.
11.   *Report on confidential enquiries into maternal deaths in England and Wales. Report on health and social subjects no. 26 1976–8.* London: HMSO, 1982.
12.   *Report on confidential enquiries into maternal deaths in England and Wales. Report on health and social subjects no. 30 1979–81.* London: HMSO, 1985.
13.   *Report on confidential enquiries into maternal deaths in England and Wales. Report on health and social subjects no. 34 1982–4.* London: HMSO, 1989.
14.   Klaus MH *et al.* Effects of social support during parturition on maternal and infant morbidity. *British Medical Journal* 1986; **293:** 585–7.
15.   Van Alten D, Eskes M, Treffers PE. Midwifery in the Netherlands. 1. The Wormerveer Study; selection, mode of delivery, perinatal mortality and infant morbidity. *British Journal of Obstetrics and Gynaecology* 1989; **96:** 656–62.
16.   Rosenblatt RA *et al.* Is obstetrics safe in small hospitals? *Lancet* 1985; **ii:** 429–31.
17.   Gaskin IM. *Spiritual midwifery.* Summertown, Tennessee: The Book Publishing Company, 1977.
18.   Morgan BM, Anaesthetic facilities. In: Chamberlain G, Gunn P, eds. *Birthplace: report of the confidential enquiry into facilities available at the place of birth conducted by the National Birthday Trust.* Chichester: Wiley, 1987.

4

There is no place for regional anaesthesia in emergency caesarean section for fetal distress

---

ARGUMENTS FOR: T. Taylor

In the mother of parliaments, important issues are frequently decided by use of a procedural motion; thus, a decision to adjourn the House can mean that this country goes to war. I have a feeling that we are also perhaps practising the same sort of procedure in this house with this motion. In this particular instance, the parliament of mothers has decided that for labour and operative delivery, epidurals are a good thing and all things general anaesthetic are a bad thing. Therefore war has been declared to prove that all things epidural must be better than all things general anaesthetic, irrespective of precise clinical situation. But what we have to do is to examine this concept critically, remembering two things.

Firstly, not all such operative deliveries take place in the ideal surroundings to which many of the theorists are so accustomed.

Secondly, it is still worth recalling that in our specialty we are still understaffed in trained anaesthetists. A workload of many extra types has been taken on in addition to the long established need to provide safe routine and emergency anaesthesia. So, we have before us a motion to an end that, although perhaps desirable, may not even be achievable.

Taken literally, this motion of anaesthesia for the purpose of emergency caesarean section must include both epidural and spinal techniques and it is therefore appropriate to deal with both. I'll consider spinal anaesthesia first.

In the British Journal of Anaesthesia in 1984, Gertie Marx[8] reviewed 126 sections for fetal distress. Anaesthesia was given by patient preference and there were 71 done under general anaesthetic and 55 by regional techniques. This is a clear majority of patient preference for general anaesthesia. Of the regionals, 33 were spinals and the other 22 had their existing epidurals extended. In the outcome there was little difference between the two groups, the most significant thing being in the one-minute Apgar score which was better for the regional techniques over the general. This of course mirrors what one would find, I think, in elective caesarean section as well as emergency. But it must be emphasised that the improvement gain was marginal.

In the discussion, Dr Marx states, and I quote: 'Frequently fetal distress is considered a contra-indication for subarachnoid block. The results of our review appear to contradict this . . .' and she continues with a passage that I think we should remember and think about. She said: 'Although the establishment of an extradural block *de novo* may be too time-consuming in the presence of fetal distress, subarachnoid blockade can be achieved in 2–3 minutes'. Finally she concludes, and I believe we should heed her words: 'Given the speed at which surgical conditions must be achieved in fetal distress, subarachnoid block emerges as the most suitable and safe method'.

In this country I don't believe there are many people who would advocate spinal as the first choice in the emergency situation, nor do I believe that most people would think it possible to achieve a successful block in 2–3 minutes, so I am not going to say much more about spinals, but I am sure it is a sound method in the hands of experts like Dr Marx and in departments like hers that are used to the method. But I don't think that the technique should be practised merely for emergency caesarean section; it should be in common usage in that hospital for other procedures. I am sure we'll find some advocates for spinals in this audience as there are some centres in this country that use it as the method of choice, but I don't believe it has found general acceptance.

Fetal distress can be defined as 'symptom complex', indicative of critical response to stress. I have taken this definition from Pernoll and Benson. It implies a potential metabolic arrangement including hypoxia and acidosis. Fetal distress may be acute or chronic and the latter I think we can ignore because most of them are due to placental insufficiency and such like causes and should not require a very urgent intervention by the obstetrician—urgent in the sense of minutes rather than hours. Regional anaesthesia in these cases is therefore possible and maybe even desirable.

Thus what we are considering, I think, in this motion is only acute fetal distress and I believe the essence of the motion is that there should be no place for epidural anaesthesia in emergency caesarean section for acute fetal distress and this is the area we should focus our attention on.

Uterine perfusion is correlated to maternal blood pressure. A fall of more than 20% in maternal baseline figures will result in a substantial reduction in uterine perfusion which will aggravate any acute intra-partum fetal distress, therefore hypotension in the mother must be avoided, whether the anaesthetic is regional or general. It is usually conceded by most anaesthetists that blood pressure falls are more likely with regional blockade, especially with a spinal, than we can confidently give in a general. This is borne out by the teaching to give large fluid pre-loads and possibly even vasopressors in regionals.

Although the incidence of maternal blood pressure fall can be and is minimised, it can and does occasionally run away, even in the best of circumstances. In poor hands, this fall can be disastrous. It is still sadly true that many (perhaps even the majority, although I can't be sure of that) anaesthetics for fetal distress are still given by juniors in training. In the circumstances of emergency caesarean section for fetal distress, the provision of an epidural performed rapidly and safely calls for an experienced anaesthetist. With the current status and number of staff employed, the regional techniques are inherently less safe than general anaesthetics. This is because of the vagaries of the so-called training that juniors receive and means that comparative competency comes sooner with the administering of a general anaes-thetic than when giving a regional block.

I think I must now quote to you from standard textbooks and I use the words of a well-known teacher and writer: Mal Morgan in Nimmo and Smith's *Anaesthesia* states that the choice of anaesthetic for caesa-rean section depends on four factors: the reason for the operation; the degree of urgency; the wishes of the patient; the skill of the operator. Later in the same chapter in the same book, he describes the technique for production of epidural anaesthesia for caesarean section and con-cludes with the words: 'This may take as long as 45 minutes'. Then he continues: '. . . even after this time, completely pain-free surgery can only be achieved in 75% of patients'.

Even allowing that the technique may be more acceptable for patients undergoing an emergency operation and is therefore less likely to fail, it is hardly an impressive success rate in a critical emer-gency situation.

If you think I'm being prejudiced, let's turn to the transatlantic textbook and I'm amused to note that Shnider and Levinson in *Miller's Anaesthesia* give the same reason for the choice of anaesthetic as Dr Morgan, and even use the same words. The Americans go on to say, and I quote: '. . . when the condition of the mother or fetus is in immediate jeopardy, caesarean section should not be delayed to ensure the adequate sensory level with either spinal or epidural block'. This directly contradicts Dr Marx. In the same section they state that among the disadvantages of epidural anaesthesia for caesarean section is the fact that the procedure is time-consuming and therefore has no place in urgent cases.

You'll have realised now that I've discussed three out of four factors given in the list above—the reason for the operation, the degree of urgency, and the skill of the operator. I have not addressed the third— the wishes of the patient. Whilst fully accepting this in the circumstances of a normal delivery, this is a very important consideration. I doubt that a mother confronted with the serious worries that the need for an urgent caesarean section brings will be in a position to be able to make a proper informed choice. Nor do I believe that a court of law in this country would think her in a position to do so. The choice must be made for her, largely by the obstetrician and anaesthetist in consultation with each other if the best conditions are to be provided at the speed which is desirable.

Thus, much of the argument I'm putting before you comes down to time, but always in the context of the degree of skill of the staff who are likely to provide the service. Why then is there so much emphasis on time? For the answer, I'll go to another standard work.

Donald, in his book *Practical Obstetric Procedures*, gives the signs of fetal distress. There is no need for me to repeat these—you are all familiar with them. But vitally, in the same passage he goes on to say quite categorically that it's too late when these signs are present. Thus what I think he's saying is that diagnosis must be made very early and the condition must almost be treated pre-emptively if the fetus is to survive undamaged.

Current litigation reinforces the view that intervention is often, for one reason or another, too late, too slow or both and let not the anaesthetist be the person be responsible for this delay. Just as an aside, you'll remember the Chief Medical Officer, Sir Donald Acheson, at a lecture he gave at the Royal College of Midwives indicating that he believed there were likely to be about 600 claims for children allegedly brain-damaged at birth in the following two years, each perhaps costing in excess of £1 million. This is over three cases per health district in the country. According to Nick Black in *The Lancet*, the cost of litigation in all specialties has risen in recent years by about 75% per annum—an incredible increase.

Defensive medicine should not only be with us, but must be actively promoted in respect of obstetrics if any money is to be reserved to treat patients in other specialities. If litigation costs escalate at the present rate, 12% of the total budget available for health care will be used to fund litigation and most of this goes on brain-damaged babies. The only alternatives are firstly, to change the law in respect of brain-damaged babies to take them out of the bracket of negligence, that is, to provide some form of no-fault compensation, or secondly, for further research to show positively which are the babies damaged at birth and determine their life expectancy exactly; that is, to make it possible to diagnose precisely the true intrapartum brain-damaged babies.

To illustrate these points that I have made, I wish to refer to some of the cases culled from the files of the Medical Protection Society. I trust I have altered them sufficiently for the hospitals and doctors not to be recognised directly because we do respect confidentiality.

Firstly, I reviewed cases of failed epidurals and have selected two of them to mention to you. I do this because failure to ensure a pain-free operation is the subject of an ever-increasing number of claims, often allied to the claim by the mother later that she had been precipitously put to sleep against her will. These events now outnumber the claims for awareness under general anaesthesia and by far outnumber the claims for failed intubation and the tragedies that they cause. Clearly, in the case of an urgent operation for fetal distress this is quite unacceptable and please note that all cases I am about to discuss were done for elective section and therefore time wasn't an enemy of the anaesthetist as it would be for an emergency situation.

In the first case I wish to recount, an explanation was given to the patient by the anaesthetist that a general anaesthetic would be induced if the epidural was not in every way satisfactory. At 11.30 am the epidural was begun and by around 12 noon there was loss of sensation tested by pinprick. Thus the patient was draped at 12.15 pm, including the insertion of skin towels into the skin around the site of incision. The first incision was made and the patient complained of pain. The anaesthetist correctly proceeded to general anaesthetic, although after the operation, the patient was found to have a complete block which lasted for some time. Thus, what we have here is not a failed epidural but one that was probably not allowed to develop fully and therefore failed surgically to anaesthetise the patient. On the other hand, the block could have been performed on this occasion on an unsuitable patient despite the fact that the block was performed at her request. Whatever the cause of this failure, this case cost £30000.

The second case, again an epidural at the patient's request, was inserted at 9 o'clock. To be fair, the anaesthetist did not regard the patient as suitable because of her personality, which is very important, and her obesity, which is also important, added to which this patient had a history of recent disc problems. However, the epidural cannula was inserted using a standard technique with bupivacaine as the local. At 9.40 am, skin testing, on this occasion by cold, revealed an incomplete block on the left hand side. Lignocaine was added as the total dose of bupivacaine given was the maximum that should be used. At 9.55 am the operation was slowly begun. Again, the patient complained of severe pain shortly after the first incision and therefore a general anaesthetic had to be induced in this case. It was said that the patient had a severe psychiatric problem as a result of her horrendous experience, and this one cost £15 000.

I have the notes of many similar cases, all showing a waiting time of up to one hour, inadequate blocks and usually reversion to general anaesthesia. Of course it is difficult to relate these statistically to the total successful cases of elective sections performed under regional blockade. But the point I'd like you to note is that the cases failed when there was time for them to be allowed to work, and lest the question be asked later, they were in some instances given by consultants, and indeed one was a private patient.

The next case is perhaps a little more relevant to the argument we are having, and therefore I'll be a little more precise in giving you the history. The patient had had two previous deliveries, was a diabetic and this was a twin pregnancy. Antenatal care had been scanty as the patient had been abroad during the early part of pregnancy. Delivery was to be at 38 weeks but this was advanced due to toxemia, as manifested by oedema, rising blood pressure and proteinuria. There was some delay in informing the spouse who was still abroad, the wife wishing him to be consulted. But at 7.30 pm an epidural was established for pain relief in labour, the membranes having been ruptured a little earlier. At that time it was hoped to effect a vaginal delivery.

By 11.15 pm there was a fall in the fetal heart rate of the lead twin, at which time the patient was fully dilated. In response to this a section was ordered. But again there was a delay, mainly due to the patient who wouldn't give her consent to the caesar without the spouse knowing, and had to be persuaded. When this was done the theatre staff and anaesthetist had to be called by taxi from the main hospital. At 35 minutes after midnight the staff arrived and the need for the operation became urgent. An argument ensued then between the patient, who wanted an epidural, and the anaesthetist, who thought that a general anaesthetic was the proper anaesthetic to give. Eventually a general anaesthetic was induced and delivery finally occurred at 45 minutes past midnight, but the first twin was very severely brain-damaged. The case was thought to be indefensible due to the delays that occurred, although many of these were of the patient's own making.

Leaving aside the question of whether the obstetric management was ideal and allowing for the fact that this case, like most others, shows more than one contributing factor, there is no doubt that the delay in this case was in the order of one hour, largely due to the anaesthetic cover provided by the health authority. But the anaesthetist also recognised that, even though there was an epidural in place, it was imprudent to proceed unless under general anaesthesia. When the operation finally got underway, the time from induction to delivery was less than seven minutes. It would have been longer if reliance had been placed on extending the epidural. Further delay would have led to damage to the second twin.

There are many other similar cases that I could recount to you, but of course time won't permit, but I do want to tell you about two more case histories because of their medicolegal importance.

The first involved a primipara and the delay, for various reasons that do not concern us here, from the first indications of fetal distress to the delivery by section under general anaesthesia was perhaps two hours. The baby was asphyxiated. In his summing up when the case came to court, the judge, after recalling the evidence he had heard from the experts, said in his view the maximum delay from diagnosis of fetal distress to delivery ought to be no more than 20 minutes, and if it were longer, it must be negligent. Personally, I think that if every obstetric unit in this country could perform within these limits, it would be miraculous. But this case demonstrates the tight time schedules under which we are forced to operate by opinions given in court. But I must emphasise that the judge derived the opinions from the evidence of experts who appeared before him. The 20 minutes quoted here must have come from the lips of the anaesthetist or obstetricians appearing and not from the mind of the judge in the case.

The second of the cases is again a baby brain-damaged due to delay, but it is the statement of **claim** which I wish to draw to your attention. This is the legal statement on which the case is based. Against the obstetrician there are five claims. The first three we can ignore—they are just routine statements about lack of care and delay from the obstetric point of view. But I want you to note the next two. Number 4 said the obstetrician permitted a delay of approximately one hour to elapse after the attempted forceps delivery and before the performance of a caesarean section. Number 5 said, 'Failed to liaise with the said anaesthetist either adequately or at all and failed to convey to the anaesthetist the urgency of the need to deliver the plaintiff'.

The claims against the anaesthetist are three.

Number 1—he failed to administer appropriate anaesthetic so as to enable caesarean section to be performed within a reasonable period of time.

Number 2—failed to comply adequately with requests from the obstetric staff to administer an appropriate anaesthetic so as to enable a caesarean section to be performed within a reasonable period of time.

Number 3—failed to appreciate the urgent need to perform a caesarean section on the plaintiff's mother (remembering it's the baby who's suing).

I think in this particular instance we should examine the history. The patient was induced at about 39 weeks because she was an elderly primipara with a systemic disease, was a heavy smoker and had shown poor weight gain. Because it was thought that she was not suitable for immediate membrane rupture, prostaglandin was inserted in order to rupture the membranes when suitable and apply a fetal scalp electrode. An epidural catheter was inserted, the membranes were ruptured at 3.30 pm with the cervix at 2 cm dilation. The liquor was clear and labour proceeded normally until at 7.45 pm, with 3 cm dilation, a scalp electrode was applied and syntocinon was started. At 11.30 pm the fetal heart was 136 and liquor clear, but at 1.55 am there was a fetal tachycardia of 170–180 with type one dips to 70 and a vaginal examination showed the patient was fully dilated. The epidural was topped up by the midwife at 2 o'clock and this was followed shortly, about 2.30, by an attempted forceps extraction by the junior in training, which failed. A decision was taken, quite correctly, and this was confirmed by the consultant, to proceed to a caesar.

The anaesthetist was in the unit, very nearby, because the anaesthetist in this hospital is actually resident in the obstetric unit and so there was no real delay in calling him. He decided to extend the epidural block before transfer to theatre. His procedure for this included a period of sitting for about 20 minutes—the patient sitting upright—during which somebody observed the fetal heart rate go down to 60. The baby was born at 3.36 am, was flat and with low Apgar scores at one, five and subsequent minutes. The delivery was 66 minutes after the failed forceps. It seems as if the anaesthetist kept the patient in the labour ward for at least 35 minutes, possibly longer, to top up the epidural. This leisurely process was compounded by delay in moving to the theatre when the patient was ready and the obstetrician was also slow with his operating. This case has recently been settled for £750 000.

Thus, in coming to any conclusion at the end of this debate, we must think in terms of the real world and leave aside notions of setting standards that are so high that they become unattainable in ordinary practice. In choosing an appropriate technique for anaesthesia for caesarean section for fetal distress, the elements which must carry the most weight are the time taken to present the patient to the surgeon coupled with the skill and experience of the anaesthetist giving the anaesthetic.

In the absence of a sure knowledge of the baby's state and realising that, if the baby exhibits any of the criteria which exist for the diagnosis of fetal distress, it may already be too late, operative delivery should be as fast as possible. The technique employed must unfailingly produce proper operating conditions for the surgeon whilst avoiding hypotension and hypoxia in the mother. With the staff and facilities available in many hospitals, this must surely mean general as opposed to an epidural or even spinal anaesthetic. I do not subscribe to the view of the learned judge that a time of about 20 minutes is the maximum that can be allowed in all circumstances before the delay becomes negligence. However, it must be rare for time to be available to allow for the initiation of a new epidural and I doubt that it would be long enough to properly top up an existing epidural. I do not believe that a spinal anaesthetic can be rushed, either.

Lastly, as I hope the cases demonstrate, there must also be some consideration of the defensive side of medicine in these circumstances. If this is not applied voluntarily and with discretion by the profession, it will certainly be imposed upon us. It is certain that this will happen with the inception of Crown indemnity run by hospital managers. The information required to do this will become available from clinical audit. I therefore suggest to you that regional anaesthesia has no place in emergency caesarean section for fetal distress.

* *

ARGUMENTS AGAINST: T. Cheek

The following outline will discuss the question: If anaesthesia is required in the presence of fetal distress, is there a role for regional anaesthesia and if so, does it provide any advantages?

Fetal distress that requires emergency delivery under anaesthesia presents the anaesthetist with a remarkable challenge. The physiological changes of pregnancy predispose to a high-risk anaesthetic. Nearly all anaesthetic drugs cross the placenta and their effect on the fetus must be considered. The parturient that requires emergency delivery is often unprepared for surgery and at risk for complications. The patient is young and often has other children and a spouse. Little margin of error is allowed to the anaesthetist yet he or she is confronted with an array of medical problems and must make speedy accurate judgements and perform with quick skill. Sometimes the speed with which anaesthesia is induced and the rapidity with which the baby is delivered may spell the difference between a neurologically intact or a neurologically damaged individual.

Despite the traditional preference for general anaesthesia in fetal distress caesarean, it is increasingly clear that rapid sequence induction is neither without major risk to the mother nor is it inevitable, as in 'I had no choice but to put her to sleep'. Regardless of the severity of fetal distress, relative indications for the choice of anaesthetic technique must be speedily considered. Recent investigation demonstrates that regional block for fetal distress caesarean is a rational alternative under most circumstances and may provide maternal and fetal advantages.

Assessment and preparation before anaesthesia during fetal distress

When notified of the need for anaesthesia in the presence of fetal distress, the anaesthetist must make a few critical assessments that will determine the anaesthetic plan.

1. Determine urgency of distress,
    a) No time,
    b) Minutes or longer,
    c) Do not unnecessarily delay surgery;
2. Presence of maternal illness;
3. Maternal airway;
4. Maternal desires if time;
5. Indications or contra-indications for regional or general;
6. Obstetrician's desires considered; anaesthetist makes final decision.

1. Determine urgency of distress:
a)   No time, a true 'stat' emergency, immediate delivery required and vaginal delivery not possible. Good examples of this situation are sustained fetal bradycardia or conditions where fetal heart rate remains less than 100 bpm the majority of the time. Fetal cardiac output is determined primarily by heart rate and sustained fetal bradycardia can result in rapid deterioration and death. Unless there is an indwelling epidural catheter with at least a T8 block level to kelly clamp and the level can be raised rapidly during preparation, general anaesthesia is usually the best choice.
b)   Rapid delivery required within 15 minutes and vaginal delivery not possible. Examples of this would be the presence of late uniform decelerations, severe variable decelerations, loss of beat to beat fetal heart rate variability or fetal pH falling below 7.21. Under these conditions there is usually time to initiate a spinal block or to increase the level of a functioning epidural catheter placed previously during labour. As a rule, it is not our practice to initiate a new epidural block under these conditions. There is no clear indication from the literature on how long the fetus will survive under these conditions. However there is no evidence that 15 minutes of preparation time will increase fetal morbidity. It is interesting to note that ACOG guidelines state, 'It should be possible to begin the operation within 30 minutes of the time that the decision is made to operate'.[1] Under no circumstances should the anaesthetist unnecessarily delay the caesarean section.

2. Determine presence of maternal illness such as infection, diabetes, pre-eclampsia, drug abuse, pre-existing medications, etc. and reconcile this information with the anaesthetic plan. For example, in the presence of severe pregnancy-induced hypertension, profound hypovolaemia is usually present and rapid spinal block under these conditions may cause a marked decrease in blood pressure that is difficult to correct. Yet a rapid sequence induction to general anaesthesia in the same patient is associated with severe cerebral and pulmonary hypertension[2] that predisposes to the common causes of maternal mortality in pre-eclampsia: cerebral haemorrhage and pulmonary oedema.

3. Evaluate maternal airway. If a difficult airway is present this will influence the choice of either the use of regional block or preparation for an awake intubation.

4. Maternal desire to be awake or asleep should be considered if there is time.

5. Indications for regional or general anaesthesia:
   a) general anaesthesia best advised:
      i) patient wants to be unconscious;
      ii) regional block not advised:
          patient refusal of regional block;
          infection over site of planned block or severe sepsis;
          uncorrected hypovolaemia;
          coagulopathy or anticoagulation;
          anatomic abnormality;
          recurrent neurological disorder;
   (iii) Extreme emergency and a functioning epidural catheter not in place:
          prolapsed cord, sustained fetal bradycardia.

Table 4.1

Factor	1973–75	1976–78	1979–81	1982–84	1973–84
Pulmonary aspiration	13	11(3)	8	7	39(3)
Anoxia (failed intubation)	7	16	8	8	39
Drug misuse	4	4	3	1	12
Apparatus	2	2	0	1	5
Epidural	2	4	1	1	8
Misc.	7	9	9	1	26
TOTAL	35	46	29	19*	129

Source: Confidential Reports on Maternal Deaths in England and Wales

b)   regional anaesthesia best advised:
  i)   patient desires to be awake at delivery;
  ii)   difficult airway predicted by exam: either regional or awake intubation;
  iii)   history of/or active asthma present;
  iv)   severe maternal hypertension present;
  v)   recent use of beta agonists: i.e. tocolysis;
  vi)   history of malignant hyperpyrexia;
  vii)   prolonged induction to delivery predicted: history previous c section.

6.   The obstetrician's desires for type of anaesthesia are considered but the anaesthetist will make the final decision.

The anaesthetist will also recall that, according to the available outcome data obtained from the Confidential Report on Maternal Mortality in England and Wales, between 1973 and 1984 78 pregnant women died due to loss of airway or aspiration and eight died of complications associated with epidural block.

There are a number of other risks to the fetus and mother associated with the rush for preparation and induction of a 'crash' caesarean section for fetal distress. The mother is fully alert and aware of the highly charged atmosphere created by the declaration of emergency, she is often hyperventilating and in great pain and almost always terrified. These conditions are all associated with a deterioration in the intra-uterine environment yet the physician has little time to alleviate these problems. Maternal fear has been shown both in primates and humans to produce fetal tachycardia, bradycardia and acidosis over a relatively short period of time.[3,4] Shnider and coworkers[5] demonstrated that severe maternal pain was associated with a 50% reduction in uterine blood flow lasting three minutes. Miller and coworkers[6] demonstrated in labouring women that sustained maternal hyperventilation was associated with a 4–5 mm decrease in fetal PO_2 Another common error in management during the rush to deliver the fetus is failure to maintain uterine displacement. The supine position during labour has been shown by Huch and coworkers[7] to produce as much as a 50% decrease in fetal PO_2. Finally, general anaesthesia for caesarean section mandates minimal amounts of induction medication and is designed to avoid neonatal drug depression. Yet this same 'light' anaesthetic is associated with marked maternal catecholamine release and may contribute to further neonatal depression from decreased uterine blood flow (Fig. 4.1).

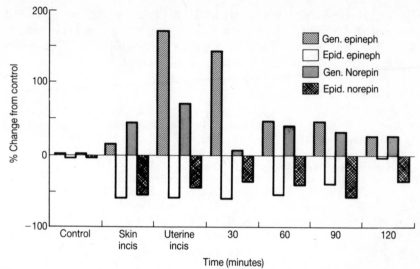

Fig. 4.1 General versus epidural anaesthetic in caesarean section. Epinephrine and norepinephrine blood levels (from Loughran PG *et al. British Journal of Obstetrics and Gynaecology*, 1986; **93:** 943)

Regional block in the presence of fetal distress

If, after appropriate assessment, the anaesthetist decides that regional block is indicated, this must be reconciled with some past misconceptions of the use of regional block in the presence of fetal distress.

1. *There is not enough time to initiate regional block in the presence of fetal distress*

a) Foresight will have a functioning epidural catheter in place. In high risk labour or those parturients in which the obstetrician detects early signs of fetal stress, the anaesthetist is consulted early to assess the patient and place a continuous epidural for maternal analgesia and as an 'insurance policy' should rapid delivery be required. The block should be maintained at T6–8 with a higher concentration of local anaesthetic than normally used for labour which will:

   i) allow caesarean section to start at once;
   ii) help prevent severe hypotension when the level is rapidly elevated to T2–4 with 3% chloroprocaine (latency 3–5 min) or 2% lidocaine.

b) If an epidural is not in place there is usually time to initiate SAB using a 22 g needle with 8–10 mg hyperbaric tetracaine, 10–12 mg hyperbaric bupivacaine or 70–80 mg hyperbaric lidocaine with epinephrine. This is usually possible in all but the most extreme emergencies.

c) Recent work by Marx and coworkers[8] prospectively looked at 126 cases of emergency fetal distress and left the choice of anaesthesia to the mother. Seventy one patients chose general anaesthesia and 55 chose regional block (33 received spinal block and 22 with catheters already in place had their block level increased).

i) Time intervals:

	Induction to skin incision	Skin incision to delivery (min)	Ut. incision to delivery (sec)
General anaesthesia (71)	67±12 sec	7.0±2.8	68.3±42.9
Regional block (55)	5.3±0.52 min	7.8±2.9	74.0±40.3

ii) Comparison of fetal blood gases (Mean ± SD)[8]:

Parameter	General Anaesthesia (A, N=71)	Regional Analgesia (B, N=55)
Scalp pH, Pre-C-section	7.204 ± .053	7.198 ± .043
U.V. pH	7.286 ± .050	7.282 ± .054
U.A. pH	7.221 ± .057	7.220 ± .053
U.V. PCO$_2$	43.1 ± 7.28	42.3 ± 6.00
U.A. PCO$_2$	49.6 ± 10.3	50.5 ± 8.23
U.V. PO$_2$	30.0 ± 8.55	26.4 ± 6.98
U.A. PO$_2$	18.0 ± 7.05	15.8 ± 5.18

A vs. B P = N.S.

iii) Conclusions: regional anaesthesia is not contra-indicated by a compromised intra-uterine environment or mild to moderate fetal distress provided that maternal hypotension is avoided or immediately treated, uterine displacement is continuously maintained, delay of delivery is not excessive ($<$10 min) and there are no other contra-indications to regional block.

2. *Regional anaesthesia contra-indicated because it will cause maternal hypotension and fetal deterioration due to decreased intervillous perfusion*
a)   Unless the mother is hypovolaemic, maternal hypotension can be avoided in most cases with appropriate uterine displacement, adequate fluid pre-load before block and intravenous ephedrine if necessary. In the event of maternal hypotension, the above recommendation and intravenous ephedrine provides rapid effective therapy. Ephedrine is not associated with decreased intervillous blood flow.
b)   There are no studies in either humans or animals that have suggested that the use of major conduction analgesia, either lumbar epidural or subarachnoid block, is associated with decreased intervillous blood flow or fetal deterioration **provided LUD is maintained and maternal hypotension is avoided**.

c)   Recent investigation by Brizgys and coworkers[9] provides evidence that maternal hypotension in the face of fetal distress is not associated with further fetal deterioration if maternal blood pressure is rapidly brought to normal.

Effect of hypotension: epidural in caesarean section[9]

Methods:
1. 583 c-sections, 38–42 weeks gestation with epidural block to t6 or higher
2. Five groups of patients
3. Local anaesthetics (% of patients):
   Bupivacaine 70%
   Chloroprocaine 24%
   Lidocaine 6%
4. Hydration 30 min pre-block 1 lit. lact. ringer
5. LUD
6. Ephedrine 25–50 mg IM within 30 min pre-block, 272 received, 311 didn't receive (not double blind)
7. Hypotension treated for 30–60 sec with further hydration and LUD. If not successful within 30–60 sec, then IV epherdrine given
8. UV and UA blood gases, 1 and 5 min Apgar scores and TSR obtained at birth.

Five patient groups: group and no.	*Ephed**		*No ephed**
1.	Elect repeat (183)	36 (35%)	34 (43%)
2.	Elect primary (39)	4 (21%)	7 (35%)
3.	Labour repeat (88)	12 (26%)	11 (26%)
4.	Labour primary (229)	10 (12%)	38 (27%)
5.	Labour, fetal dist primary (44)	8 (50%)	8 (28%)

*Number and % having hypotension defined as systolic BP <100 or fall >30%.
P=NS between epherdrine and non ephedrine groups.

Group 5, fetal distress:

Umbilical arterial values (n=35)

	pH	*PO_2*	*PCO_2*	*BD*
Normotensive	7.20±0.01*	14.1±1.1	55.3±1.5	6.6±0.7**
Hypotensive	7.19±0.02	13.6±2.0	58.7±3.9	6.3±0.9

*$P < 0.05$ Lower than normotensive values in groups 1, 2, and 4
**$P < 0.05$ Greater than normotensive values in groups 1–4
P = NS Group 5 *normotensive* vs *hypotensive*

Conclusions:
1. Hypotension is seen *less* in patients *in labour*.
2. LUD, pre-hydration with 1.0 litre BSS, and prophylactic ephedrine may *not* prevent hypotension, especially in the non-labouring parturient.

3. IM ephedrine prophylaxis is *not* effective in preventing hypotension.
4. Rapidly treated maternal hypotension is *not* associated with significant deterioration in either stressed or non-stressed fetuses.

d)   Other studies in humans, often using patients as their own controls, have indicated that intervillous blood flow and fetal status are unchanged or improved in high-risk patients receiving regional block:

i)   Hypertensive: Jouppila R *et al.: British Journal of Obstetrics and Gynaecology* 1979; **86:** 969 (epidural);

ii)   Pre-eclampsia (severe): Jouppila R *et al.: Obstetrics and Gynecology* 1982; **59:** 158 (epidural);

iii) Diabetes: Datta S *et al.: Anesthesia and Analgesia* 1982; **61:** 662–665 (spinal).

Important points to remember: major conduction block for fetal distress

a)   Anticipate the need and increase the use of epidural block in suspected high-risk labouring patients. Should emergency caesarean section be required, this will:
1. provide for an orderly, smooth transition to anaesthesia for caesarean section;
2. avoid the highly charged atmosphere of the rush to 'crash' induction;
3. decrease the chance for physician error due to fear, anger or excessive speed. There may be some evidence that this 'error factor' contributes to morbidity, loss of airway control and aspiration.

Anaesthetic maternal mortality incidence

Elective caesarean section   1/10,000
Emergency caesarean section   1/2000
(Pakter J *et al.* Maternal and perinatal mortality. In: Marx GF, ed. *Clinical Management of Mother and Newborn.* New York: Springer Verlag, 1979: 241–264)

b)   Emergency caesarean for fetal distress declared:
1. Surgeon accurately assesses time allowed and clearly communicates this to the anaesthetist;
2. Assure IV non-dextrose solutions, high F_1O_2 >50% till birth, maternal and fetal monitors, LUD until birth, Bicitra 30 ml p.o.
3. Extend functioning epidural or initiate spinal anaesthesia if time allows.
4. *Do not delay surgery in the presence of dire distress, e.g.*
i) Unremitting fetal bradycardia;
ii) Prolapsed cord;
iii) Severe abruption—maternal hemorrhage.
5. General anaesthesia, if chosen, should be induced with a qualified assistant only when surgeon prepared, patient draped and suction

up, usually by rapid sequence induction unless airway anatomy is difficult, then either awake intubation or regional block.
6. Surgeon cuts only when airway assured.

Medicolegal Implications of Regional Block and Fetal Distress

Recent reports from the ASA closed malpractice claims database[10] found that payment proportions were similar between obstetric (53%) and non-obstetric (59%) claims. Median payments for OB claims were significantly greater ($203 000) compared to non-OB claims ($85 000). Obstetric claims involving general anaesthesia were more frequently associated with severe injuries and resulted in higher payment than did claims involving regional anaesthesia. Newborn brain injury was the second leading complication. Of the 17 cases of newborn brain injury attributed to anaesthesia, four had general anaesthesia and 13 regional as the primary technique. Brain damage due to delay of anaesthesia occurred once in each group (25% for GA, 8% RA).

The majority of RA complications associated with newborn brain damage were caused by maternal convulsion (9). This evidence does not support the notion that the 'extra time' required for regional block will leave the anaesthetist at greater risk for malpractice suits for neonatal brain damage. It has also been shown above[8] that induction to delivery intervals under regional block for fetal distress in a large series can average 11–12 minutes. This is well within the limits set by ACOG standards that state 'it should be possible to begin the operation within 30 minutes of the time that the decision is made to operate for fetal distress'.[1] It should be emphasised that once a decision is made for regional block, the anaesthetist should not perseverate beyond one or two quick attempts at a spinal block nor should incision be delayed to wait for an indwelling epidural level to rise. This is not a time to be 'macho' or to 'prove your stuff'. If regional block is not adequate by the time the surgeon is ready with patient draped, knife in hand and suction running, progression to general anaesthesia should be immediate. In the rare (~1 in 3–4000) instance where the maternal airway is extremely difficult, awake intubation must be considered.

Of similar concern is the effect of maternal hypotension/uterine hypoperfusion on the distressed fetus during anaesthesia induction regardless of technique. It is important to note that under general anaesthesia, maternal hypertension is not always associated with adequate uterine perfusion. Indeed, catecholamine induced uterine hypoperfusion has been observed in animal models and in some human studies under general anaesthesia. Recent work shown above[9] has demonstrated that rapid correction of maternal hypotension is not associated with significant metabolic deterioration in the stressed fetus.

The diagnosis of fetal distress often leads to a sudden and often artificially tense environment that may lead to haste-induced and unnecessary maternal/fetal injury. Anaesthetists who encounter complications during emergency general anaesthesia induction can no longer hide behind the excuse, 'I had no other choice'. The use of regional block is a rational and in many cases a preferable alternative and should be included among the accepted anaesthetic techniques used with fetal distress.

REFERENCES

1. Frigoletto FD, Little GA, *et al. Guidelines for perinatal care.* American Academy of Pediatrics and American College of Obstetricians and Gynecologists, 1988.
2. Hodgkinson R, Husain FJ, Hayashi RH. Systemic and pulmonary blood pressure during caesarean section in parturients with gestational hypertension. *Canadian Anaesthetists Society Journal* 1980; **27:** 389–94.
3. Cofer DE, Huber CP. Heart rate response of the human fetus to induced maternal hypoxia. *American Journal of Obstetrics and Gynecology* 1967; **98:** 320.
4. Morishima HO, Pederson H, Finster M. The influence of maternal psychological stress on the fetus. *American Journal of Obstetrics and Gynecology* 1978; **131:** 286–90.
5. Shnider SM, Wright RG, Levinson G, Roizen MF, Wallis KL, Rolbin SH, Craft JB. Uterine blood flow and plasma norepinephrine changes during maternal stress in the pregnant ewe. *Anesthesiology* 1979; **50:** 524–7.
6. Miller FC, Petrie RH, Arce JJ, Paul RH, Hon EH. Hyperventilation during labor. *American Journal of Obstetrics and Gynecology* 1974; **120:** 489–95.
7. Huch A, Huch R, Schneider H, Rooth G. *British Journal of Obstetrics and Gynaecology* 1977; Suppl. 1: 1.
8. Marx GF, Luykx WM, Cohen S. Fetal-neonatal status following caesarean section for fetal distress. *British Journal of Anaesthesia* 1984; **56:** 1009–13.
9. Brizgys RV, Dailey PA, Shnider SM, Kotelko DM, Levinson G. The incidence and neonatal effects of maternal hypotension during epidural anesthesia for cesarean section. *Anesthesiology* 1987; **67:** 782–6.
10. Chadwick HS, Posner K, Caplan RA, Ward RJ, Cheney FW. A comparison of obstetric and non-obstetric anesthesia malpractice claims. *Anesthesiology* 1991; **74:** 242–9.

5

Accidental dural taps must be treated by immediate bloodpatching

ARGUMENTS FOR: I. Findley

Introduction

Accidental puncture of the dura is the commonest cause of prolonged morbidity following epidural analgesia for labour or anaesthesia for caesarean section in obstetrics. The ensuing headache causes great misery to the patient and her family as well as the staff caring for her.

The reported incidence of unintentional dural puncture varies from 0.3 to 2% or even higher. The occurrence varies with the experience of the operator and is, as expected, higher in teaching institutions. The attention to a careful technique is paramount in the prevention of dural taps. The incidence of incapacitating severe headache in young obstetric patients following puncture with a size 16 or 18 gauge epidural needle is extremely high (70–80%).[1] The implications of prolonged hospital stay for the patient are important as is the burden on the provision of obstetric beds in the light of present financial restraints. Leakage of cerebrospinal fluid through the hole in the dura leads to the headache by stretching of pain sensitive structures anchoring the brain, such as blood vessels and the tentorium.[2] The headache is diagnostically worse on standing and relieved in the supine position. Loss of cerebrospinal fluid in the obstetric patient, who may already be dehydrated from fluid restriction in labour, can have serious complications such as cranial nerve damage, and subdural haematomas have been reported.[3,4]

Epidural bloodpatches are well established since Gormley first reported them in 1960[5] as treatment of post-spinal headache. Di Giovanni established the safety and efficacy of epidural injections of autologous blood for post-lumbar puncture headache in animal studies and in humans. His report includes five cases of successful immediate prophylactic bloodpatch following accidental dural puncture. **Immediate**, i.e. minutes after the tap, and **prophylactic**, i.e within 12 hours of delivery, will be considered synonymously for the purposes of this discussion.

Conservative management

The traditional management of unintentional dural puncture includes:

1. nursing supine;
2. regular analgesics;
3. high fluid intake;
4. laxatives;
5. abdominal binding.

Lying flat is very distressing for the obstetric patient who needs to look after her new baby. The supine position will relieve the headache but not prevent it developing.

High fluid intake of 3–4 litres/day is usually encouraged. However, there is no evidence that it increases the production of cerebrospinal fluid. It certainly increases the production of urine and makes the patient more aware of her disability by having to go to the toilet frequently.

Epidural infusion of balanced salt solutions (1–1.5 litres/24 hr)[7] decreases the incidence of dural tap headache from >70% to 12–30%, but has the disadvantage of confining the patient to bed.

Intravenous caffeine sodium benzoate[8] is effective in alleviating the headache but gives temporary relief and only delays the definitive treatment, which is epidural bloodpatch.

Epidural bloodpatching

The efficacy of epidural bloodpatching with autologous blood is well proven for treatment of established dural puncture headache. Most epidural bloodpatches in this country are performed more than five days after the puncture.

Ostheimer[9] in 1974 reported a prospective study undertaken by the Society for Obstetric Anaesthesia and Perinatology on the effectiveness and safety of epidural bloodpatches. Out of 185 patients, 182 or 98.4% had complete and permanent pain relief within 24 hours. There were no serious or permanent complications. Selwyn Crawford in this country advocated therapeutic epidural bloodpatching and described this technique.[10] By increasing the volume of blood injected from 10 ml to up to 20 ml, he improved the success rate of therapeutic bloodpatching from 89% to 99%.[10]

Laboratory and clinical studies[12,13] have shown no long-term adverse effects of blood injected into the epidural space. Animal studies on goats showed that the clot gradually organises and after three months the histological picture is the same as that following a simple epidural. Restricted spread of analgesia following epidural bloodpatch has been reported[14] and it was suggested that the clot might have caused fibrous tethering of the dural to the wall of the spinal canal, causing a physical obstruction to the spread of local anaesthesia in the epidural space. However, in a longer term study, others[15] have shown that epidural analgesia may be impaired in patients who have had a previous dural tap. The chance of poor analgesia is 35–40% in this group and is not related to the application of an epidural bloodpatch.

Contra-indications

There have been no reported untoward serious sequelae following provision of epidural bloodpatches. The commonest complaint is a sensation of fullness or bruising in the back. Parasthesia may occur and prevents the injection of the whole 20 ml of blood. The backache usually disappears after two days but patients should be warned before the procedure.

Pyrexia is an absolute contra-indication to autologous blood-patching because of risk of bacteraemia and epidural abscess formation.

Prophylactic bloodpatching

The use of bloodpatch in the management of headache following dural tap is well established, being safe and effective. Dural puncture with a large epidural needle is almost certain (80% chance) to produce a severe incapacitating headache which, although self-limiting and unlikely to lead to morbidity if treated conservatively, causes great misery to the patient. The reluctance of the medical profession to prevent the headache is thus difficult to understand since many patients require a bloodpatch later anyway.

By applying a prophylactic patch after every accidental dural puncture, a small number (20%) of patients would receive an unnecessary bloodpatch. Also there is concern that epidural analgesia will be patchy and inadequate. Loeser *et al.*[16] suggested that the failure rate of early patching, i.e. within 24 hours, was as high as 71% compared to 4% for patches done after 24 hours. They injected only 10 ml of blood whereas it is now accepted that 17–20 ml is required for better success.

Quanor[17] reports seven non-obstetric patients in whom the accidental dural puncture was treated with a bloodpatch within 15 minutes by injection through the epidural needle. Some of these patients received satisfactory epidural analgesia via a catheter following the bloodpatch. None of the patients developed headache.

Immediate prophylactic bloodpatch was studied in the prevention of post-dural puncture headache after spinal anaesthesia for extracorporeal shockwave lithotripsy.[18] This group had a very high incidence of headache (45%). In the treated group the incidence was reduced to 8.3% without any serious implications by immediate bloodpatching following the dural puncture.

Obstetric patients with complication of unintentional dural tap often require further analgesia, usually epidurally, for labour and delivery. Few studies of the use of the epidural catheter for prophylactic injection bloodpatch are available. Ackerman[19] reported a 100% success rate after injection of 15 ml autologous blood via the epidural catheter in just six patients even though the blood was not deposited at the site of puncture because the catheter was inserted at a higher lumbar level.

Recently Colonna-Romano,[20] in a controlled study of 39 patients, showed that the incidence of headache following unintentional dural puncture with an epidural needle was reduced from 80% to 21% by prophylactically injecting 15 ml of autologous blood after delivery and before removing the epidural catheter. In this way, some patients (20%) do receive a useless bloodpatch and indeed some patients receive an unnecessary patch (20%). The success rate is not as high as for a late therapeutic patch, but 60% do benefit and avoid the misery of the incapacitating headache. Injecting through the epidural catheter already placed avoids the risks of another epidural and indeed another dural tap.

The main concern about an epidural bloodpatch after delivery is that of placement of infected blood into the epidural space leading to abscess formation. There is often a temporary bacteraemia at the time of vaginal delivery so it would seem prudent to wait about 12 hours after delivery before administering the bloodpatch. Blood cultures are taken at the same time as the blood for patch. Intravenous broad spectrum antibiotics may be considered before administration of the bloodpatching. Pyrexia is the obvious contra-indication to a prophylactic bloodpatch.

In Summary

The risk of developing a dural puncture headache following an unintentional dural tap with an epidural needle in the obstetric population is extremely high (80%). In most cases the conservative treatment is unsatisfactory and only delays effective treatment. Prophylactic bloodpatching via the epidural catheter avoids the risk of another epidural. The technique is safe and effective and should be available to all mothers who want it after explanation of the risks and benefits.

Further studies on the effectiveness and safety of epidural blood-patch for dural tap are required probably on a multicentre basis as the experience obtained in any one hospital is limited.

* *

ARGUMENTS AGAINST: A. P. Jarvis

The treatment suggested in the title of this chapter has been on many minds for some time. The concept of treating accidental dural taps, or inadvertent dural punctures (IDPs), by bloodpatching with an autologous epidural blood patch (AEBP) has been around since the early 1960s, yet there is still great debate as to when, in a time sense, AEBPs are best employed. There is also great debate as to whether AEBPs are the best prophylactic technique to use against the complications of IDPs, of which the post-dural puncture headache (PDPH) is the most common and best known. In order to answer this question, we need to answer several other questions before a final, informed decision can be made. The first question is a very simple one; that is, whether IDPs need to be treated at all, and if so, the next question is whether this is immediate or delayed. The final question is whether the primary method of treatment should be an immediate AEBP or not.

Must accident dural taps be treated?

We should all ask ourselves, why must IDPs be treated, and what are the risks of not treating them? We all know of the severe nature of the headaches associated with IDPs. Indeed, the first description of a post-dural puncture headache (PDPH) was well documented by Bier as long ago as 1899, in his essay on cocainising the CSF. In his article, Bier[21] states that:

> . . . I felt severe pressure on my skull upon standing up too fast from a chair, accompanied by slight dizziness. All these symptoms disappeared as soon as I laid down in a horizontal position but came back after I stood up . . . I had to go to bed and remain there for nine days because on standing up all the symptoms described returned again.

As we can see from just this one reference, PDPHs do respond to time, this being the rationale for one of the modes of treating PDPHs, that is bedrest and reassurance. The headache may be either occipital with radiation to the back of the neck, or bifrontal with radiation to behind the eyes. It is usually dull in nature when lying down, becoming intense when the patients sit up. Other symptoms commonly associated with the headache include nausea and vomiting, photophobia, dizziness, tinnitus and depression. This latter phenomenon is more commonly and thus more importantly seen in the post-partum population. Every effort must therefore be taken to keep the frequency of occurrence in this group of patients to a minimum. The headache normally goes by the fifth to seventh day; indeed 80% will have gone by the end of the second week, although there have been reports of it lasting much longer[22,23].

Both Bromage[24] and Crawford[25] have stated that not all IDPs progress to cause a headache, a figure of 70–80% getting headaches being most commonly quoted. This incidence is likely to be more severe in the obstetric patient compared to the non-obstetric, because of the episodes of 'pushing' and the tendency to dehydration that is seen during the peripartum period. The incidence of headaches, and to some extent their severity, are also directly related to the size of the dural tear, the size of the tear being related to the size of needle causing it. If we talk about a 16 g epidural needle then a figure of around 70% is correct, but if we are looking at 20 g needles, for example when performing myelography or discography, in these cases following a deliberate dural puncture, then the incidence of headache falls approximately 20%. This figure falls still further if one uses 26 g needles, the size of needle currently suggested for obstetric spinal anaesthesia. In this particular field of anaesthesia an incidence of greater than 0.5% would be considered too high by some (Table 5.1).

When we consider the severe nature of the headache following an IDP it is quite reasonable to state that some form of preventive measure needs to be taken to decrease the incidence of this complication. The likelihood of an IDP occurring is dependent on two things: firstly the skills of the operator, and secondly the co-operation of the patient. In the teaching hospital maternity environment, the incidence of IDPs has been quoted as being up to approximately 2%.[25] Although this incidence can be kept to a minimum through close supervision of trainees, there will always be a small number of accidental punctures

Table 5.1   Incidence of Dural Puncture Headache v Gauge of Needle (from literature review)

Gauge	%
16	60–70
18	25
20	10–15
25	1–1.5
26	0.2–0.5

occurring each year. It should be stressed that trainees are not the only personnel who have IDPs; it has been pointed out many times that the occasional epiduralist will have an equally high incidence, that is until his skills are reinforced by practice. In view of the iatrogenic nature of this problem, it should be the policy of every unit to have a protocol for the management of IDPs and their complications.

It is also important to remember that headaches are not the only complications to follow an IDP. Less common but equally as important are the various cranial nerve palsies particularly the VI (60%) and VII (30%)[22] of reported cases, loss of hearing,[22,26] subdural haematoma,[3,27,28] and there is one report suggesting that convulsions may occur as a result of an IDP.[29] So again, we have very good reasons for treating inadvertent dural punctures actively.

IDPs—How sould we manage them?

There are three lines of approach in managing IDPs. Firstly, there are those methods designed to prevent or reduce the incidence of complications following an IDP. An alternative approach is to wait and see if a PDPH occurs and then treat it actively. However, a third line is more commonly taken, that of prophylaxis against the development of PDPHs and then active management of them if they do occur.

Prevention of PDPHs

Over the years many techniques of preventing the development of PDPH following an IDP have been suggested (see Table 5.2). These range from simple bedrest to what we would now regard as quite bizarre ideas. Many of the ideas suggested were to increase cerebral

Table 5.2   Suggested methods of treating IDP's/IDPH's

Psychological support and reassurance of recovery
Bedrest in head-down position
Icebag to head
Oral fluids
IV fluids isotonic/hypertonic
Abdominal binders
Sedation/analgesics
Caffeine sodium benzoate/thiophyllines
Catgut dural plugs
Formal repair of dural puncture
Epidural bloodpatches immediate/delayed
O_2/CO_2 inhalation
Epidural injections/infusions
Subarachnoid injections
5% ethyl alcohol

blood flow and thus increase CSF production, the inhalation of carbon dioxide being an example of this. Another technique increasing CSF production was suggested by Deutsch in 1952,[30] namely the use of intravenous infusions of 5% ethyl alcohol in distilled water, the logic behind this idea being dilation of the vessels in the choroid plexus and increased CSF yield.

In 1930, as part of his Masters degree, Nelson[31] suggested that placing 3 cm catgut plugs into the dural tear would close the hole and so stop CSF leakage. He reported that his technique decreased the incidence of PDPHs from 17.2% in the controls to 4.9% in those with catgut plugs. It is interesting to note that those anaesthetists who regularly use a continuous spinal technique, in which an epidural catheter is deliberately placed in the CSF, will say that their incidence of PDPHs is very low, indeed much lower than would be expected for the size of dural puncture. Their argument is that the presence of the catheter sets up a local tissue reaction that seals the dural puncture site when the catheter is removed. Maybe the concept of placing catgut in the dural puncture hole is not as bizarre as first thought.

All of these methods, however, have had their problems and have not stood the test of time. Those methods of preventing PDPHs commonly considered in current practice are: use of small needles, prevention of CSF loss (i.e. no pushing with delivery), abdominal binders, general body hydration (orally or intravenously), epidural injections or infusions of saline, and immediate autologous epidural blood-patches.

Needle size: As mentioned previously, the smaller the needle the lower the incidence of PDPHs (see Table 5.1). It should be remembered, though, that multiple dural penetrations with small needles increase the incidence of PDPH compared to a single penetration. It has also been shown that penetrating the dural longitudinal fibres with the needle bevel parallel to them decreases the likelihood of PDPHs compared to a fibre cutting approach.[32,33]

Prevention of CSF loss: Any increase in CSF pressure will tend to increase the loss of fluid through the dural puncture. The act of pushing produces CSF pressure greater than that in the epidural venous plexuses, so increasing the CSF loss. In the obstetric patient it has been suggested that a limited duration of the second stage should be permitted with an early intervention of a forceps delivery if necessary. In order to facilitate this, good epidural analgesia should be established at a higher intervertebral level. There is, however, some evidence that pushing in the second stage does not influence the incidence of PDPHs,[34] and some authors question the medicolegal problems that might arise with an assisted forceps delivery,[35] particularly if this technique is used with all patients in whom an IDP has occurred.

Epidural infusions of saline, following the successful resiting of an epidural catheter, have been advocated by several authors[2,36,7] as a means of reducing the amount of CSF leaked through the dural puncture. Following Moir's description of the technique in 1971, Crawford[7] reported his success in preventing the development of PDPHs by the administration of 1–1.5 litres of Hartmann's solution into the epidural space. Of the 18 patients studied, 11 had no headache, five had mild headaches and the other two had severe postural headaches. It was noted that this latter group did not receive the full course of treatment, and it has been suggested that the rate of infusion and the duration of infusion may very well affect the overall success of this technique. Current opinion suggests that infusions of at least 1 litre of n/saline over 24–36 hours, via the epidural catheter, reduce the incidence of PDPHs significantly, perhaps in up to 85% of cases,[1] thus making this a useful technique in trying to prevent the occurrence of PDPHs following IDPs.

Hydration: Most of the treatments for PDPHs are mainly directed to returning the CSF pressure to normal. Rehydration is important in two respect. Firstly if the patients are dehydrated, then any technique designed to increase CSF production will be less effective. Secondly, as part of the nature of the problem, patients are confined to bed feeling worse for wear and dehydration does not help matters. It has been recommended that a fluid intake of 3000 ml per day be administered, this being either orally or, in the presence of nausea and vomiting, intravenously.[37,38] DDAVP has also been used in order to maintain adequate hydration,[39] although it remains an experimental technique at the present time.

Increasing CSF pressure: Increasing the CSF pressure is a mode of therapy aimed at reducing the compensatory cerebral vasodilation seen after CSF loss, thus decreasing the likelihood of PDPHs developing. Increased abdominal pressure will increase epidural vein pressures and thus CSF pressure, by compression of the dura in the abdominal region. Abdominal binders[40] are effective in this way but are not commonly used due to the discomfort of wearing them.

Another method of compressing the dura and subsequently increasing CSF pressure is the placement of a large volume of saline or blood into the epidural space, i.e. an epidural injection of saline or an autologous epidural bloodpatch. Epidural saline injections of 60 ml have been shown to increase CSF pressure and to reduce the incidence of headaches from 76.5% to 12.5%.[41] However, more lasting results have been reported following an AEBP, this being due to the dual action of instilling blood into the epidural space, namely increasing CSF pressure by dural compression, and sealing the dural puncture site by clot formation. Recently there have been numerous reports concerning the effectiveness of immediate AEBPs, some suggesting that they work, others that they are inconsistent in their success rates.[1,2,16,42] Loeser[16] in his article found a very high failure rate (71%) when the prophylactic bloodpatch was performed less than 24 hours after the initial dural puncture (see Fig. 5.1). Part of the mechanism for failure might be related to the continued fluctuations in cardiovascular parameters and CSF pressures seen immediately following delivery. These changes are thought to prevent the sealing action of the AEBP from working completely. It appears therefore that, in general terms, the earlier that an AEBP is sited following an IDP then the lower the likelihood of it working.

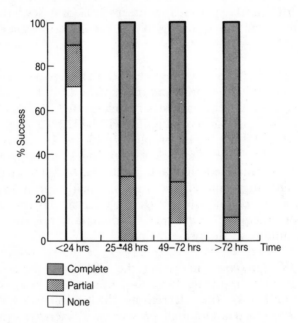

Fig. 5.1 Time versus success rate for epidural bloodpatch (from Loeser, *Anesthesiology* 1979; **49:** 148)

Treatment of PDPH

The currently accepted method of treating a PDPH once it has developed is that of initial bedrest, good hydration and simple analgesia for 2–3 days, followed by a 20 ml AEBP if the headache persists. It has long been the standard teaching that, following both spinal anaesthesia and an IDP, all patients should be nursed on their back for 24 hours. The reasons for this are that bedrest would decrease CSF loss but recently there have been several reports[6,42] that suggest that this practice is unnecessary; indeed one of them[6] suggests that early mobilisation decreases the incidence of PDPH. Hydration, as previously mentioned, is important, as is the administration of regular simple analgesics, although prophylactic systemic analgesia is unlikely to be effective. Epidural bloodpatches were first described in 1960 by Gormley[5] and subsequently, following Di Giovanni's papers,[11,12] became the 'gold' standard for treating PDPHs. The volume of 20 ml is critical to the incidence of success as Crawford reported in 1980.[1]

More recently there have been several question marks raised against the long term safety of instilling blood into the epidural space. In 1983, Rainbird and Pfitzner[14] showed radiographic evidence of fibrous bands being formed across the epidural space following a previous epidural bloodpatch, and the subsequent failure to achieve an adequate epidural block. Crawford[10] in 1985, reporting on his experiences with AEBPs, showed that in one of the 17 patients who had a repeat epidural following a previous epidural bloodpatch, there was a mechanical block at the level of T10 that prevented the follow-up epidural working properly.

Discussions with both orthopaedic and neurosurgical colleagues who have a particular interest in spinal surgery have elucidated that blood in the epidural space and its subsequent clot and fibrosis formation may cause some of the chronic backaches that they see (personal communications). It is now routine that in most spinal surgery absolute haemostasis at the end of the procedure is sought and that a fat pad is placed over the nerve roots and dura in order to reduce the amount of fibrosis around the nerve roots.

It has been postulated that the fibrotic process, with subsequent tethering of nerve roots, leads to the long-term failure of surgery in some of these patients. Di Giovanni in 1972[12] clearly showed the fibrotic nature of a small volume of blood when injected into the epidural spaces of goats. The histological findings showed that the fibroblastic reaction reached a peak at three weeks with the collagen formation measuring five times the thickness of the dura in those animals given blood, whereas in the control animals the reaction was minimal. At three months the resulting 'scar' was the same thickness as the underlying dura. Di Giovanni also noted that in some control animals there was some 'scarring' as a result of the trauma of simply placing a needle into the epidural space. It should be noted that Di Giovanni's work was using a much smaller volume of blood (2 ml) than is currently being used, so his findings (that there was no evidence of long-term complications with AEBPs) may not be as conclusive in view of current clinical practice of using large volume AEBPs.

Other complications of autologous epidural bloodpatching are better known, namely the risks of infection (from blood contamination), the risk of a repeat dural puncture, backache,[9,13] headache[9,13] tinnitus,[44] and abdominal cramps.[9] In 1973 and 1975 there were two papers that reported temporary radiculitis[45,46] that lasted for about two weeks, the proposed mechanism for the pain being initially irritation of the nerve root by the injected blood and secondly traction on the nerve root as a result of clot retraction.

Alternative methods of treating PDPHs

Caffeine

Caffeine sodium benzoate (CSB) has been used very successfully over the years as a means of treating PDPHs. In order to understand its mode of action, the pathophysiology of PDPHs needs to be reviewed.

It has been taught for many years that the cause of the headache following a dural puncture is the loss of CSF from the puncture site. Indeed, losses of up to 50 ml have been reported.[47] The loss of CSF results in a decrease in intracranial volume that allows the meninges to stretch and put traction on the falx, communicating blood vessels and nerves, this traction causing the classic pain of a PDPH. More recently, it has become clear that this classic description is not correct. The fundamental cause for PDPHs is agreed to be the leak of CSF from the dural puncture site, leading to a subsequent fall in intracranial pressure (ICP). In response to the fall in ICP, it has been proposed that there is compensatory vasodilation of cerebral vessels and increased cerebral blood flow.[45,46] This combination causes stimulation of the pain fibres that surround the cerebral vessels as they dilate, thus causing pain. Clinically the pain is greater in the sitting position, due to the ICP being significantly lower, than when patients are lying down. With a lower ICP there is a greater degree of vasodilation seen and a corresponding increase in pain.

Caffeine is a cerebral vasoconstrictor and has been shown to increase cerebral vascular resistance and decrease cerebral blood flow.[45] By causing a decrease in the degree of cerebral vasodilation, the pain of PDPHs is cured. This mechanism of action means that there should be a further fall in ICP following caffeine administration. This fact has been known since it was first reported in 1931.[48] If the mechanism of PDPHs was purely one of mechanical traction on the intracranial structures, then any further reduction in ICP should make things worse and any technique that increases ICP, for example jugular vein occlusion, should improve the headache. Both these assumptions are incorrect, i.e. caffeine[49] with its decrease in ICP cures PDPHs and jugular occlusion makes things worse.[50]

Clinically, intravenous infusions of caffeine sodium benzoate containing 250 mg caffeine and 250 mg sodium benzoate have been shown to relieve PDPHs in up to 70% of patients.[8,51,52,53] Various authors have used different volumes of infusion in order to try to improve the success rate, but there appears to be little difference between the lowest (2 ml) and the largest (2 litres). One study showed a significant decrease in pain, as assessed using a visual analogue scale.[8] This study demonstrated that pain levels decreased after the first two courses of treatment (see Fig. 5.2). The conclusion was that caffeine was effective in curing PDPHs following an IDP in approximately 60% of cases and that no more than three doses should be given, as any more were unlikely to improve this figure. The only reported side effects of caffeine administration for the relief of PDPHs have been transient dizziness and mild flushing.[49] However there is one report of postpartum seizures[53] temporally related to the management of a PDPH with caffeine and an AEBP. Following this report it has been recommended that caffeine be avoided in patients who might be susceptible to seizures, i.e. epileptics and pre-eclamptics.

A currently suggested protocol for the administration of intravenous caffeine is detailed in Table 5.3. The volume of administration is not critical, as previously mentioned, and should be reduced if clinically indicated. The rationale behind the use of a large volume of infusion is that most patients suffering with a PDPH tend to be dehydrated from lack of fluid intake.

Table 5.3 Protocol for Intravenous Caffeine Sodium Benzoate

1. Confirm presence of PDPH
2. 500mg CSB in 1 litre 0.9% saline IV over one hour
3. Repeat (2) after eight hours
4. Assess headache; if cured, no further action; if PDPH persists, repeat (2) at 16 hours
5. If PDPH still present at 24 hours or returns, consider AEBP

Summary

We have now discussed the reasons for treating inadvertent dural punctures, and have confirmed the need for some form of prophylactic management of them in order to prevent the undesirable complications, of which the post-dural puncture headache is the most important. Various prophylactic measures have been proposed, the use of epidural infusions and perhaps a well-managed second stage of delivery being the most effective. It is my belief that because of the potential long-term complications of autologous epidural blood-

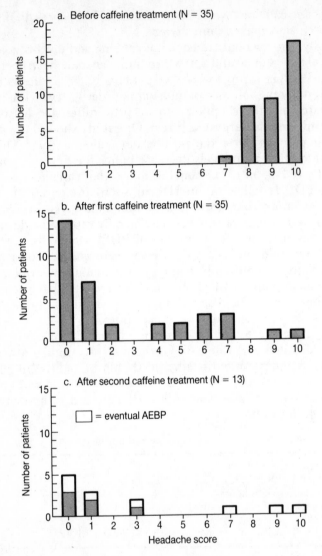

Fig. 5.2a-c Distribution of pain scores (0=nil, 10=maximum) (from Jarvis *et al.* *Regional Anesthesia* 1986; **11**: 42)

patching, namely fibrosis of the epidural space, it is wrong to use this method as a prophylactic treatment. Prophylaxis, by the very nature of the term, involves giving a treatment to patients who may not develop the problem in the first place. In view of this, I feel that only techniques guaranteed to be complication-free should be used. AEBPs do not in my mind fall into this category.

So the answer to the question, 'Should accidental dural punctures be treated by immediate bloodpatching' is, 'No, they should not'. The correct answer, I suggest, is to prevent the occurrence of complications following an accidental puncture with epidural infusions of saline, to keep the patients well hydrated and analgesed. If a post-dural puncture headache subsequently develops, then I suggest that three doses of caffeine sodium benzoate are given as outlined in Table 5.3, and only then, if the PDPH persists, should the use of an AEBP be considered.

REFERENCES

1. Crawford JS. Experiences with epidural bloodpatch. *Anaesthesia* 1980; **35:** 513–15.
2. Brownridge P. The management of headache following accidental dural puncture in obstetric patients. *Anaesthesia and Intensive Care* 1983; **11:** 4–15.
3. Edelman JD, Wingard W. Subdural hematomas after lumbar dural puncture. *Anesthesiology* 1980; **52:** 166–7.
4. Jack TM. Post-partum intracranial subdural haematoma: a possible complication of epidural analgesia. *Anaesthesia* 1979; **34:** 176–80.
5. Gormley JB. Treatment of post-spinal headache. *Anesthesiology* 1960; **21:** 565–6.
6. Thornberry EA, Thomas TA. Posture and post-spinal headache. *British Journal of Anaesthesia* 1988; **60:** 195–7.
7. Crawford JS. The prevention of headache consequent upon dural puncture. *British Journal of Anaesthesia* 1972; **44:** 598–600.
8. Jarvis AP, Greenwalt JW, Faeraeus L. Intravenous caffeine for post-dural puncture headache. *Regional Anesthesia,* 1986; **11:** 42.
9. Ostheimer GW, Palakniuk RJ, Snider SM. Epidural bloodpatch for post-lumbar-puncture headache. *Anesthesiology* 1974; **41:** 307–8.
10. Crawford JS. Epidural bloodpatch. *Anaesthesia* 1985; **40:** 381.
11. Di Giovanni AJ, Dunbar SB. Epidural infections of autologous blood for post lumbar puncture headache. *Anesthesia and Analgesia,* 1970; **49:** 268–71.
12. Di Giovanni AJ, Galbert MW, Wahle WM. Epidural injection of autologous blood for post-lumbar-puncture headache: additional clinical experiences and laboratory investigation. *Anesthesia and Analgesia* 1972; **51:** 226–32.
13. Abouleish E, de la Vega S, Blendinger I, Tiong-oen T. Long-term follow-up of epidural bloodpatch. *Anesthesia and Analgesia* 1975; **54:** 459–63.
14. Rainbird A, Pfitzner J. Restricted spread of epidural analgesia: case report with a review of possible complications. *Anaesthesia* 1983; **38:** 481–4.
15. Ong, BY, Graham CR, Ringaert KRA, Cohen MM, Palahniuk RJ. Impaired epidural analgesia after dural puncture with and without subsequent bloodpatch. *Anesthesia and Analgesia* 1990; **70:** 76–9.
16. Loeser EA, Hill GE, Bennett GM, Sederberg JH. Time vs. success rate for epidural bloodpatch. *Anesthesiology* 1978; **49:** 147–8.

17. Quanor H, Corbey, M. Extradural bloodpatch—why delay? *British Journal of Anaesthesia* 1985; **57:** 538–40.

18. Sengupta P, Bagley G, Lim M. Prevention of postdural puncture headache after spinal anaesthesia for extracorporeal shockwave lithotripsy: an assessment of prophylactic epidural bloodpatching. *Anaesthesia* 1989; **44:** 54–6.

19. Ackerman WE, Colclough GW. Prophylactic bloodpatch: the controversy continues. *Anesthesia and Analgesia* 1987; **66:** 913.

20. Colonna-Romano P, Shapiro BE. Unintentional dural puncture and prophylactic epidural bloodpatch in obstetrics. *Anesthesia and Analgesia* 1989; **69:** 522–3.

21. Bier A. Experiments from cocainising the spinal cord. *Dtsch Z Chir* 1899; **51:** 391.

22. Vandam LD, Dripps RD. Long-term follow up patients who received 10,098 spinal anesthetics. *Journal of the American Medical Association* 1956; **161:** 586–91

23. Abouleish E. Epidural blood patch for the treatment of chronic post lumbar puncture cephalgia. *Anesthesiology* 1978; **49:** 291–2.

24. Bromage PR. *Epidural analgesia.* Philadelphia: WB Saunders, 1978.

25. Crawford JS. Lumbar epidural block in labour: a clinical analysis. *British Journal of Anaesthesia* 1972; **44:** 66.

26. Lee CM, Peachman FA. Unilateral hearing loss after spinal anaesthesia treated with epidural patch. *Anesthesia and Analgesia* 1986; **65:** 312.

27. Welch K. Subdural haematoma following spinal anaesthesia. *Archives of Surgery* 1959; **79:** 49–51.

28. Pavlin DJ, McDonald JS, Child B. Acute subdural haematoma—an unusual sequlla to lumbar puncture. *Anesthesiology* 1979; **51:** 338–40.

29. Vercauteren MP, Vundelinckx GJ, Hanegreefs GH. Postpartum headache, seizures and bloodstained CSF: a possible complication of dural puncture. *Intensive Care Med* 1988; **14:** 176–7.

30. Deutsch EV. The treatment of post spinal headache with intravenous ethanol: a preliminary report. *Anesthesiology* 1952; **13:** 496–500.

31. Nelson MO. Post puncture headaches: a clinical and experimental study of the cause and prevention. *Archives of Dermatology* 1930; **21:** 616–27.

32. Greene HM. Lumbar puncture and prevention of post-puncture headache. *Journal of the American Medical Association* 1926; **86:** 391–2.

33. Franksson C, Gordh T. Headache after spinal anesthesia and a technique for lessening its frequency. *Acta Chir Scand* 1946; **94:** 443–54.

34. Ravindran RS, Viegas OJ, Tasch MD, Cline PJ, Deaton RL, Brown TR. Bearing down at the time of delivery and the incidence of spinal headache in parturients. *Anaesthesia and Analgesia* 1981; **60:** 524–6.

35. Rubin AP. Obstetric anaesthesia. In: Kaufman L, ed. *Anaesthesia review 3.* Edinburgh: Churchill Livingstone, 1985.

36. Craft JB, Epstran BS, Coakley CS. Prophylaxis of dural puncture headache with epidural saline. *Anaesthesia and Analgesia* 1973; **52:** 228–31.

37. Moore DC. *Anesthetic techniques for obstetrical anesthesia and analgesia.* Springfield: Charles Thomas, 1964.

38. Zuspan RP. Treatment of postpartum postspinal headache. *Obstetrics and Gynecology* 1960; **16:** 21–6.

39. Cowan JMA, Durward WF, Harrington H, Johnson SH, Donovan B. DDAVP in the prevention of headache after lumbar puncture. *British Medical Journal* 1980; **280:** 240–4.

40. Kunkle EC, Ray BS, Wolff HG. Experimental studies on headache, analysis of the headache associated with changes in intracranial pressure. *Arch Neurol Psych* 1943; **49:** 323–58.

41. Usubiaga JE, Usubiaga LE, Brea LM, Goyena R. Epidural and subarachnoid space pressures and relation to post spinal anaesthesia headache. *Anesthesia and Analgesia* 1967; **46:** 293–6.

42. Palahnuik RJ, Cumming M. Prophylactic blood patch does not prevent post lumbar headache. *Canadian Anaesthetists Society Journal* 1979; **26:** 132–3.

43. Jones RI. The role of recumbency on the prevention and treatment of post-spinal headache. *Anesthesia and Analgesia* 1974; **53:** 788–96.

44. Glass PM, Kennedy WF Jr. Headache following subarachnoid puncture: treatment with epidural blood patch. *Journal of the American Medical Association* 1972; **219:** 203–4.

45. Sechzer PH. Post spinal anaesthesia headache treated with caffeine. Part 11: Intracranial vascular distention a key factor. *Curr Therap Res* 1979; **26:** 440–8.

46. Cass W, Edelist G. Post spinal headache: successful use of epidural blood patch 11 weeks after onset. *Journal of the American Medical Association* 1974; **227:** 786–7.

47. Pickering GW. Lumbar puncture headache. *Brain* 1984; **71:** 274–80.

48. Denker PG. The effect of caffeine on the cerebrospinal fluid pressure. *American Journal of Medical Science* 1931; **181:** 675–81.

49. Sechzer PH, Abel L. Post spinal anaesthesia headache treated with caffeine: evaluation with demand method. Part 1. *Curr Therap Res* 1978; **24:** 307–12.

50. Tourtellotte WW, Haerer AF, Heller GL, Somers JE. *Post lumbar puncture headaches*. Springfield: Charles Thomas, 1964.

51. Harrington TM. An alternative for spinal headache. *Journal of Family Practice* 1982; **15:** 172–7.

52. Clark RB. Conduction anesthesia. *Clinical Obstetrics and Gynaecology* 1981; **24:** 601–17.

53. Bolton VE, Leicht CH, Scanlon TS. Postpartum seizure after epidural blood patch and intravenous caffeine sodium benzoate. *Anesthesiology* 1989; **70:** 146–9.

6

Gaining experience of general anaesthesia for caesarean section is a justification for maintaining the rate above 20%

ARGUMENTS FOR: A. Spence

I shall begin by saying something about the philosophy of the recognition of training programmes.

It is clearly necessary for bodies such as the College of Anaesthetists, or any body concerned with quality assurance, to set standards for training, firstly in the best public interest and secondly which are attainable within a working practice. An example relates to the use of extradural block analgesia in labour. Five or six years ago there was much discussion at what was then the Faculty of Anaesthetists as to what was needed for this particular component of training. There is danger in trying to determine a 'norm', because numbers become more important than the quality of the training. It is important, in deciding what the quality of a programme of training is, to gauge what is adequate in relation to the opportunities available.

On the subject of extradural analgesia in labour there were many members of the Faculty of Anaesthetists at that time who were keen to press for an increase in the number of extradural services in this country and to produce that pressure through a training requirement. However, a central body such as that College of Anaesthetists should resist such pressure. I remember one hospital group that did not offer extradural analgesia. I knew the hospital well and could understand why that was so. It would have been very dangerous to impose the service by central dictat. It would be far more sensible to say that if experience is to be gained, those in training should be seconded somewhere else.

What do the college regulations say? Not a lot. Essentially, all that the *'Requirements for General Specialist Training'* states is that there should be enough experience to practise general and regional anaesthesia and analgesia for obstetrics under appropriate supervision and that that should have been achieved after completion of appropriate general professional training. The basic criterion is what is possible in a particular setting.

This leads to the motion itself and the figure of 20%. I must state straight away that I have a problem with this figure and would prefer not to defend it as a number, but rather as a concept. My consultant colleagues in Edinburgh obstetric anaesthesia provided me with the figure for the Simpson Memorial Pavilion. The Pavilion involves a big service and we have taken the figures from the years between 1979 and 1989. The number of deliveries for these years respectively are very similar: 4700 and 4600.

The rate of epidural block, primarily for relief of pain, is unchanged over that period and stands at 28% of all these deliveries. There is a change in the use of subarachnoid block: 12 in 1979 and 116 in 1989. This is less than happens in some other services and it is important to note that it is only two cases a week.

The rate of caesarean section is also almost unchanged: 13% in 1979 and 14% in 1989. But the ratio of elective to emergency caesarean section is altered. There are more emergency sections as a proportion now than occurred ten years ago. If you take nerve block over general anaesthetic, the ratio was 1.3:1 in 1979, 5:1 in 1989. The same ratio for emergency caesarean section is also changed although the change is less marked. It was 0.6:1 in 1979 and 2:1 in 1989.

I do not consider these figures to be untypical in a large service. I think that in terms of the shift away from the use of general anaesthesia, compared with many of the smaller hospitals, it represents more of a front-line position than an average for the UK. The point is that although over the ten years there was a shift, it is not as marked as the motion would presuppose. I am not unduly worried. I don't think the implied problem exists or at least, it has not yet arrived.

But let's suppose it had arrived; if so, we would clearly have an ethical dilemma based on the supposition that there will never be a situation in which we would need to resort to general anaesthesia for operative obstetric delivery.

Is there anything special about the pregnant woman as a candidate for general anaesthesia making it necessary for those in training to gain special experience in obstetrics? I presuppose that an audience such as this believes there are differences; I certainly do. If the issue of numbers became really critical, then maybe teaching simulators could be designed to provide the experience. However, one thing I do not urge, and nobody should urge, is that there be an artificial rearrangement of the best therapies for patients in order to meet the needs of training.

Over the years we have invested the practice of obstetric anaesthesia with a mystique that in many instances scares people presenting as novices or in training. Even if this mystique were only applied to general anaesthesia in obstetrics, there would still be a strong case for offering adequate experience if only to allow the trainee to discover that the practice of obstetric anaesthesia is not so difficult.

Finally, what about 20%? As it stands in a large service like the Simpson Memorial Pavilion and the Royal Infirmary of Edinburgh, there are less than four cases a week available for elective caesarean section with a general anaesthesia rate of 20%. I would say that this is about the minimum for people to feel adequately comfortable in what they are doing. Thus, while I hold to my view that we shouldn't defend a number for its own sake, I think that 20% is at about the lower limit of what is desirable.

* *

ARGUMENTS AGAINST: F. REYNOLDS

Professor Spence and I are probably more in accord than in opposition. I too would not like to put a precise figure on a desirable rate of general anaesthesia for caesarean section. It is more in the philosophy of our approach to the problem that I think we differ. He suggests that an epidural service ought not to be introduced for the benefit of trainees. I too would be horrified at the idea that anyone would introduce an epidural service for the benefit of trainees; I would rather it were introduced for the benefit of patients. One must not lose sight of the fact that in the long run every policy we adopt must be for the benefit of patients. We do not carry out procedures in order to train junior staff; we train juniors to carry out what we believe to be the best procedures for patients.

The first anaesthetic that I was taught to use was ether, and ten years later I found myself distressed that young anaesthetists no longer knew how to give an ether anaesthetic and I used to wonder how, ethically, I could select a patient to undergo this unsatisfactory and uncomfortable experience in order to train junior staff. I gave up. But the problem of training junior staff to give general anaesthesia for caesarean section is, as Professor Spence has implied, as yet a rare one. We in our ivory towers consider that we may be presiding over the demise of general anaesthesia for caesarean section, but what is the position in the country as a whole? In the South East Thames region, for which I can speak, 12 districts were able to tell me the epidural rates for caesarean section as well as for deliveries as a whole (Fig. 6.1). In the remaining districts, epidural rates were not high. It is quite clear that in the South East Thames region, with the exception of only one health district, the problem is much more how to train

EPIDURALS IN SE THAMES REGION

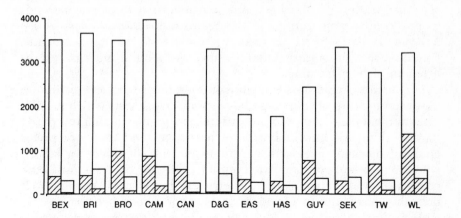

Fig. 6.1 Epidural rates in 12 Districts in the South East Thames Region. Left hand column: number of deliveries; Right hand column: number of caesarean sections. Hatched areas: number of epidurals.

juniors to give **epidural** rather than general anaesthesia both for deliveries and for caesarean sections, and this I submit is where our energies should be directed. With the current fashion for rotations of junior staff at every level, there is currently no difficulty in picking up the appropriate experience in different types of anaesthesia in different hospitals.

The crucial problem is to provide adequate training for all junior staff in the safe and successful administration of epidural analgesia. There are many reasons for advocating this, and epidural block has so many advantages over general anaesthesia for caesarean section that I think it an appalling idea that any woman should be denied these advantages. Firstly the question of unplanned awareness. Readers may recall a case[1] in which a woman had suffered pain and awareness under so-called general anaesthesia for caesarean section and it was declared that the anaesthetist was not negligent because anaesthesia had been conducted correctly. Well, it may not be negligent but it certainly contravenes the Trade Descriptions Act! I fail to see how anybody could advocate preserving any form of management which can have such a disastrous result though the procedure may be carried out entirely correctly.

There are of course disadvantages to both techniques and I think it essential for this debate that they should be weighed up, although they are well known. From the mother's point of view, as well as unplanned awareness, general anaesthesia carries the risk of gastric aspiration, failed intubation, uterine relaxation, damage to teeth, lips and tongue and, as is fashionable nowadays, there is no shared experience for mother, father and baby. Post-operatively there is the danger of recurarisation (as has been reported following tubocurarine and. more recently, pancuronium in the *Reports on Confidential Enquiries into Maternal Deaths*), gastric aspiration, sore throat, pain, nausea and vomiting, slow mobilisation and possibly late bonding and slow establishment of breastfeeding.[2]

Opponents of epidurals will point out that they are time-consuming. To overcome this, of course, we have spinal anaesthesia which may be essential in a busy unit or for an extreme emergency in an unprepared mother. I myself have a horror of headaches and therefore prefer epidural blockade for elective sections and for all women in labour who are at risk of operative intervention. This, of course, requires the co-operation of midwives and obstetricians but works extremely well once they have faith in a good epidural service. For emergency caesarean section, extending a block can occupy as little time as it takes to prepare a woman for surgery and once she is ready the time which would otherwise need to be devoted to pre-oxygenation, injection of thiopentone and suxamethonium, application of cricoid pressure, laryngoscopy and passing the tracheal tube, blowing up the cuff, attaching the anaesthetic equipment, testing for leaks and correct tube placement, can all be saved.

The next disadvantage, the possibility of hypotension and a poor response to haemorrhage, I cannot argue with. However, in larger centres in the States where the commitment to epidural analgesia is even greater than it is in my unit, I have heard epidural analgesia may even be advocated in the presence of anterior placenta praevia. Next, there may be intrapartum nausea which can be dealt with by maintaining the blood pressure and giving anti-emetics, substernal pain which can be cured by epidural opiates, and the risk of dural puncture which can be reduced to less than 1:300 with good training. Local anaesthetic toxicity may result from accidental intravenous injection but this complication would appear to be commoner in the US than in this country. Serious sequelae and late neurological complications may result from clinical error and can be avoided by careful attention to detail. It is far easier to train staff not to give the wrong drug than it is to train them to intubate successfully on every occasion.

However, it would perhaps be preaching to the converted to dwell any longer on the relative advantages to the mother of epidural rather than general anaesthesia for caesarean section. But what about the baby? One factor that is often overlooked is that, provided the maternal blood pressure is maintained, regional anaesthesia provides definite advantages for the baby without any disadvantages.[3] Once consumers really get wind of this, I suspect it may become negligent not to use regional analgesia. The advantages to the baby probably lie in avoiding general anaesthesia (though any sedation resulting in the baby is of course readily reversible) and in the improved maternal placental blood flow that results from sympathetic blockade, which can be particularly advantageous in pre-eclampsia.[4] General anaesthesia is not able to produce the appropriate selective vasodilatation within the uteroplacental bed. Some years ago Marx and her colleagues,[5] and more recently the Cardiff team,[6] showed that Apgar scores are significantly better in babies born by caesarean section under epidural blockade than with general anaesthesia. Moreover the neurobehavioural status of the baby is also enhanced provided there has been no hypotension,[7] and the final arbiter, perinatal mortality, also comes down in favour of epidurals[8,9].

But what of maternal death? Over the 15 years 1970 to 1984 there were 123 deaths associated with general anaesthesia and eight with epidurals, and this over a period when my calculations suggest more women would have received epidurals than general anaesthesia. Moreover, the deaths associated with epidural block are such as would largely be avoidable by careful training rather than necessitating increased skill, as is the case with deaths due to general anaesthesia.

Is general anaesthesia so very much more difficult in the obstetric patient than in any other surgical emergency? Professor Spence touched on this point. It is true the same technique will be used in both situations, namely a rapid sequence induction. It is true also that intubation may on average be somewhat more difficult in the obstetric patient. This should not mean we should go out of our way to try and give more general anaesthetics; rather we should ensure that juniors are taught to give the *best* technique, by which, as Andrew Doughty has said many times, it is possible to teach them to **stay out of trouble**. Yet many juniors today lack this sort of experience and it is precisely in this area that our efforts in training should lie. What right have we to subject a woman to an unnecessary risk to pursue an undesirable technique? More careful and assiduous training in epidural and spinal blockade is what is needed. There can be no justification for giving general anaesthesia to a woman on any other than exclusively medical grounds.

REFERENCES

1. Brahams D. Caesarean section: pain and awareness without negligence. *Anaesthesia* 1990; **45:** 161–2.
2. Morgan BM, Aulakh JM, Barker JP, Reginald PW, Goroszeniuk T, Trojanowski A. Anaesthetic morbidity following caesarean section under epidural or general anaesthesia. *Lancet* 1984; **i:** 325–30.
3. Reynolds F. Effect on the baby of regional blockade in obstetrics. In:

Reynolds F, ed. *Epidural and spinal blockade in obstetrics*. London: Bailliere Tindall, 1990.

4. Jouppila P, Jouppila R, Hollmen A, Koivula A. Lumbar epidural analgesia to improve intervillous blood flow during labour in severe preeclampsia. *Obstetrics and Gynecology* 1982; **59:** 158–61.

5. Marx GF, Luykx WM, Cohen S. Fetal–neonatal status following caesarean section for fetal distress. *British Journal of Anaesthesia* 1984; **56:** 1009–13.

6. Evans CM, Murphy JF, Gray OP, Rosen M. Epidural anaesthesia for elective caesarean section: effect on Apgar score and acid-base status of the newborn. *Anaesthesia* 1989; **44:** 778–82.

7. Abboud TK, Naggappala S, Murakawa K, *et al.* Comparison of the effects of general and regional anesthesia for cesarean section on neonatal neurologic and adaptive capacity scores. *Anesthesia and Analgesia* 1985; **64:** 996–1000.

8. David H, Rosen M. Perinatal mortality after epidural analgesia. *Anaesthesia* 1976; **31:** 1054–9.

9. Ong BY, Cohen MM, Palahniuk RJ. Anesthesia for cesarean section—effects on neonates. *Anesthesia and Analgesia* 1989; **68:** 270–5.

7

Epidural opiates should be abandoned in obstetric patients

ARGUMENTS FOR: S. Woods

Controversies in obstetric anaesthesia

The use of epidural opiates in obstetrics has become a cause for concern. There have been a growing number of reported cases in which the use of extradural opiates has led to respiratory depression. Fortunately, so far this has always been recognised and treated in time, but the danger of serious consequences, even of death, remains if diagnosis should be delayed. This danger is exacerbated by the difficulties at present faced by the NHS with the consequent shortage of staff and inadequate monitoring facilities. In spite of this the use of epidural opiates in obstetric analgesia is becoming more popular, even in cases where their use is not justified. A review of all the arguments for and against suggests that the use of epidural opiates cannot be justified in the present state of knowledge and the existing medical environment.

Need for improved pain relief in labour

Maternal distress in labour is often compared indiscriminately with physical pain, for which the obvious answer is sufficient analgesia. Nevertheless, there are enormous variations in individual responses to labour, arising from differences in personality and in the ability to deal with a situation of great potential stress. Each individual's analgesic requirement must therefore be assessed and the giving, by a midwife, of universal fixed doses of pethidine irrespective of a woman's size or pain threshold is bad obstetric management. Indeed, it may lead to disorientation and failure to co-operate at delivery.

Reassurance by the obstetrician that the labour will be conducted by one sympathetic midwife and within a certain period of time will do much to alleviate the need for analgesia. Even so, there will still be a need for analgesia in almost all cases. The presence of the anaesthetist in the labour ward supervising analgesia is essential to good pain management. When opiates are properly titrated according to the mother's requirements, or when a mother can control her own analgesia, then we have a more satisfactory situation. The end result is that the mother is happier and more co-operative, resulting in more economical use of the opiate.

Extradural analgesia with bupivacaine has little effect on the awareness of the mother, does not depress the baby's respiration, and produces complete pain relief. Much can be done to reduce the local anaesthetic side effects of weakness, hypotension and poor expulsive efforts.

The need for improved pain relief for post-operative caesarean section

In cases of caesarean section post-operative management is often badly done once the woman returns to the ward. The inconvenience of giving a controlled drug on the ward has induced some anaesthetists to set up an infusion in the recovery room. Those who can may use their patient-controlled analgesic (PCA) machines.[1,2] In any event the need for opiates is short-lived. Milder oral analgesics are usually sufficient after 24 hours. More use of the non-steroidal anti-inflammatory drugs should be made, one suppository lasting for 24 hours with good effect.

Historical review

When in 1973 Pert and Snyder[3] discovered specific opiate receptors and later pinpointed their presence in the substantia gelatinosa of the spinal cord,[4,5,6] this provoked a flood of clinical reports. Wang in 1979[7] reported a research study in the use of intrathecal morphine in patients with malignancies. He pointed out the exceptionally long-lasting analgesic properties of this opiate. Behar and Olswang *et al.*[8] 28 days later used the same drug epidurally in ten patients and testified likewise. Cousins *et al.*[9] reported favourably on the use of epidural pethidine. Enthusiasm escalated and as a result there were many case reports and reviews of the pharmacology[10,11,12,13,14] and of their clinical relevance.[15,16,17,18] They showed that the prolonged analgesia was related to the cerebrospinal fluid (CSF) concentration, and that analgesia existed without any motor, sensory or autonomic deficits. This type of pain relief they called 'selective spinal analgesia'.

Advantages of epidural opiates

The pain relief produced by extradural opiates with their protracted duration of action, and lack of any motor, sensory or autonomic impairments was indisputable.[7,8,9] The possibility of using a vast range of opiates and the existence of a specific opiate antagonist was hopeful. Obstetric anaesthetists were naturally encouraged by the prospect of producing complete, long-lasting analgesia, free from the side effects of systemic opioids and local anaesthetics.

Disadvantages of epidural opiates

Four months after Wang's initial report in 1979,[9] Scott and McClure[19] reported two cases of delayed respiratory depression following epidural pethidine. Subsequent acknowledgements followed.[20,21,22,23] The respiratory depression reported[22,23] happened many hours after the administration of small doses of the opiate.

Mode of action

A certain quantity of an epidural dose of opiate will diffuse across the dural sheath, enter the CSF and then the nervous tissue to assimilate with the specific opiate receptors within the spinal cord. It is this direct transfer of epidural administration that represents its pharmacokinetic advantage over other systemic avenues. Diffusion depends on the physical nature of the membrane—the dura—and the physicochemistry of the different drugs. Permeability is indirectly proportional to the width of the dura. It declines in thickness from the cervical to the sacral region. The molecular weight and shape as well as the lipophilicity is important when considering receptor access and binding.

Dural transfer

The amount of drug available for dural transfer can be calculated but pregnancy markedly affects the transfer of drugs, since it raises the venous pressure in the extradural veins and so will result in an increase in flow through the azygos vein (Fig. 7.1). This would result in an increased rate of systemic absorption of drug with less drug available for transfer across the dura. This may explain the relative failure of extradural opiates in pregnancy. The clinical effect from extradural opiates results from direct dural transfer and from systemic absorption.

The circulation of the cerebrospinal fluid

There is rostral motion in the CSF. Pulsatile movements in the CSF occur simultaneously with respiration and cardiac systole. Events such as coughing or straining can grossly affect CSF activity.[16] Studies

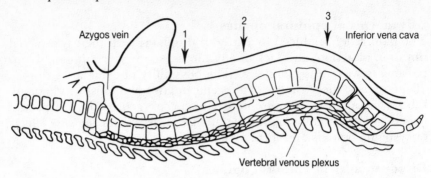

Fig. 7.1 Venous drainage of the epidural space into the inferior vena cava (IVC) via the azygos vein. Compression of IVC at 1, 2 or 3 results in rerouting of venous flow by internal vertebral plexus (epidural) veins to azygos vein. Increased intrathoracic pressure is transmitted to epidural veins and may result in increased flow up the portion of internal vertebral venous plexus that is protected within the vertebral body (modified from Bromage PR. *Epidural analgesia.* Philadelphia: W B Saunders, 1978, with permission of the publisher)

in man using 10 mg of extradural morphine showed a progressive cephalad spread to the trigeminal areas. This is absolutely in keeping with the hypothesis of upward transfer of the drug by the CSF tide. Potentially fatal delayed respiratory depression occurs in much the same way. The use of caution in relation to spinal opiates is essential.

Predicted benefits of extradural opiates in obstetrics
It was hoped that epidural opiates would produce:

1. prolonged analgesia without any motor or sensory loss;
2. prolonged analgesia without any hypotension (since no sympathetic block);
3. no respiratory depression.

Side effects
It was not surprising that epidural opiates produced some of the well-known opiate side effects of:

Nausea and vomiting

Vomiting occurs not infrequently[24] but it is worrying as it may be causative in the development of respiratory depression by encouraging rostral spread of the opiate in the CSF. This happens because of the increase in intra-abdominal pressure associated with vomiting.

Pruritus

Itching occurs with practically all epidural opiates, usually confined to the head and neck. Data comparing the incidence of itching is non-existent. Histamine is not always involved in itching; it occurs even with fentanyl, which does not release histamine from mast cells. Antihistamines have little effect. It is antagonised by naloxone. It is thought to be central in origin and related to the dose of the drug. It is a consistent complication in labour.

Urinary retention.

It is the most troublesome complication of epidural opiates. The effect of morphine on the bladder has been known for some time. Catheterisation may be required after therapeutic doses of morphine, and it is suggested that central effects of opiates may make patients inattentive to stimuli arising from the bladder.

Respiratory depression

Respiratory depression is present when the normal stimuli of hypoxia or hypercapnia persistently fail to excite the respiratory centre of the brain to respond normally. Temporary alterations in the pattern or rhythm of breathing should act as warning signs, although sleep, per se, may produce similar patterns of apnoea and hypoventilation. It cannot be adequately stressed that hourly respiratory rate checks may not pick up either the premonitory or the full-blown signs of respiratory failure. It is because of this fact that the use of monitoring equipment must be continuous, and as such, it must be comfortable.

Many methods of measuring ventilation are impractical, for example strain gauges and inductance plethysmograph. Transcutaneous carbon dioxide electrodes are inaccurate. Pulse oximetry, to measure oxygenation, is comfortable and accurate over 70% saturation. Blood gases tensions are used despite the time delay and the non-continuous invasive nature of the technique. The measurement of the respiratory rate intermittently may be a simple one, but it is also a simplistic one. The relationship between the arterial oxygen tension, carbon dioxide tension and respiratory rate is unreliable. It is possible to maintain a normal respiratory rate in the presence of hypoxia or hypercapnia.

Spinal opioids, having penetrated the dura relative to their physicochemical properties, enter the cerebrospinal fluid. They enter the opiate receptors of the spinal cord and travel cephalad with the CSF flow or become metabolised. Respiratory depressant concentrations may reach the chemosensitive areas of the brain stem either in the bloodstream or in the CSF.

Dural transfer of opioid depends on the molecular weight and the lipophilicity of the drug. Fast onset of analgesia is synonymous with lipophilicity to a great extent. It is this lipophilicity that confers the advantages of fentanyl and sufentanil, now being tried, not very successfully, in labour.

As has been described, whilst in the epidural space, the opiates may enter the epidural veins where they are swept away in the azygos vein because of the increased venous pressure, due to inferior vena cava compression in late pregnancy. This would leave less drug available for transfer across the dura into the spinal cord. Except for morphine, most opiates readily cross the dura if the concentration gradient is favourable, and enter nervous tissue or the circulation. As a result the CSF concentration of these drugs reduces very quickly with a corresponding reduction in cephalad spread. It is the lack of lipophilicity of morphine which increases its concentration in the CSF and leaves it more prone to travel rostrally to produce delayed respiratory depression.

Bromage *et al.* provided evidence for this in giving morphine 10 mg to ten healthy volunteers and noting signs of dermatomal spread to the trigeminal area in six hours in all ten subjects, as evidenced by loss of sensation to pinprick and ice, which implied cephalad spread to the brain stem. Coughing, vomiting and artificial ventilation, all common in the post-operative patient, may increase the cephalad spread in the CSF circulation.

Table 7.1

Opioid	Lipid solubility	Molecular weight	pK (25 C)	Partition coefficient
Morphine	1.42	285	7.9	1.42
Meperidine	38.8	247	8.5	38.8
Methadone	116	309	9.3	116
Fentanyl	813	336	8.4	813
Alfentanil	126			
Sufentanil	1778	386	8.0	1778
(−) Lofentanil cis-oxalate		408	7.8	1450
Endorphin		3300	—	—

Predisposing factors contributing to respiratory depression

Advanced age is put forward as one of the factors contributing to respiratory depression. There have, however, been reports of respiratory depression in the young.[25,26] The lipophobic drug morphine has been implicated most frequently, but reports of respiratory depression with all the opiates have occurred. Lack of tolerance may make a subject more susceptible to the side effects. Because of this many centres give one extradural injection of diamorphine for post-operative pain. Caution should be used in giving extradural opiates in the presence of other sedative drugs such as diazepam droperidol or given by other routes. What may be a potentially serious predisposing factor in labouring mothers is the use of the valsalva in the second stage, which may accelerate cephalad spread of the drug. Similarly with coughing and vomiting. Use should be made of smaller doses of extradural opiates because of the serious reports with large doses.

Factors compounding respiratory depression[27]

Pre-existing chronic obstructive airways disease in patients who are given epidural opiates may compound the abnormal parameters of respiratory depression. Upper airways obstruction, because of a deviated septum or a small mandible, may potentiate any respiratory depression. Many normal people have sleep apnoea, and this may also tip the balance in an already compromised woman. Obesity may produce similar problems. It is almost certain that obstetric women are protected somewhat more than similar non-pregnant women, because of their increased respiratory effort in late pregnancy.

Simultaneous use of parenteral narcotics and sedatives is often a factor implicated in respiratory depression. The longer term use of large doses of hydrophobic opiates which are repeated as a bolus dose, or which are given by infusions, appear to put a person more at risk of developing respiratory depression.

There is a much higher incidence of respiratory depression after intrathecal administration than after epidural administration.

Prevention of respiratory depression

McCaughey and Graham[28] have pointed out the dangers of the supine or head-down position, and have advised that women who have had epidural opiates should be nursed in a semi-sitting position. They feel that this affords a certain degree of protection, as their studies showed an increase of respiratory depression in women nursed flat. The use of smaller doses of lipophilic drugs would certainly help to prevent respiratory depression. Patient selection in terms of age and fitness is important. Prophylactic use of naloxone infusions has met with a general lack of enthusiasm, because of its tendency to reduce the analgesia and because it was not effective in avoiding but only in reducing the side effects. The avoidance of simultaneous use of parenteral opiates, sedatives or other centrally depressant drugs is essential, as well as avoidance of larger doses of hydrophobic opiates. For post-operative caesarean sections, one post-operative dose of a lipo-philic opiate appears to be quite adequate.

Avoidance of raised intrathoracic or intra-abdominal pressure may be more possible in theory than in practice in the obstetric patient.

Incidence of respiratory depression

The overall incidence has been stated at 0.09–3%,[29,30] but a true figure is not possible to evaluate. Many case reports have occurred in patients receiving parenteral narcotics in the presence of epidural opiates, and may have been in high-risk patients. Nevertheless respir-atory depression occurs in the absence of any identifiable factors. Many papers point out the safety of epidural opiates in the obstetric patient for post-operative pain, because of the lack of risk factors. However a recent publication has made us aware that it still occurs when no risk factors are present.

Many[31,32,33,34] have attempted to determine the incidence of respir-atory depression in caesarean section by monitoring the degree of somnolence and the respiratory rate intermittently. Their studies were all done with epidural morphine 5 mg. The incidence of respiratory depression was determined by a respiratory rate of 10 minutes or less and the results varied. Although the incidence was relatively low, periods of apnoea or hypoventilation may have occurred. How many of these patients had significant CO_2 retention but normal respiration rates is unknown.

Although the incidence seems to be small, there remain many un-reported cases; a true estimate is not possible.

Naloxone and its shortcomings

Naloxone is a pure opioid antagonist. It will reverse respiratory de-pression produced by an agonist or a partial agonist. Larger amounts of naloxone are required in the case of partial agonists. After IV injection some effects of naloxone can be seen in 1–2 minutes with a duration of 45–90 minutes. The onset of action of naloxone after intramuscular injection is 15 minutes. Naloxone given to the mother just prior to delivery appears to be undesirable. Birth is a stressful process for the fetus and the endorphins produced possibly aid the fetus in withstanding the stress. Therefore, naloxone may be detri-mental in fetal welfare.

The usual dose recommended in narcotic overdose is 10 μg per kilogram initially intravenously, repeated at 2–3 minute intervals as needed. Doses as large as 8 mg may be needed. Infusions of 4 mg of naloxone in 1000 cc of 5% dextrose can be used. A healthy adult may require 100 ml per hour. Patients, including newborns of mothers who are or may be physically dependent on narcotic or narcotic-like compounds, may experience withdrawal when given naloxone. There are reports of induced hypotension. Other reports have supported this naloxone-induced catecholamine-releasing theory. Sudden cardiac arrest occurred in two healthy young women within minutes of intravenous administration of naloxone in order to antagonise the effects of narcotic drugs during anaesthesia. It can be inferred that along with the abrupt increase in blood catecholamines, hypoxaemia may have contributed to the fatalities.

Effectiveness of epidural opiates in labour

Unfortunately, in labour, morphine has too slow an onset of action. Pethidine, similarly, is of no use as it requires very large doses to be effective. Interestingly, it lasts longer when given intramuscularly than when given epidurally.[35,36] Butorphanol has been used in America, and was found to produce extreme somnolence.[37] Only fentanyl[38,39,40,41] and sufentanil,[42,43,44] when used in conjunction with bupivacaine, have been shown to produce early improved and longer lasting analgesia than bupivacaine alone. However, alone they are unpredictable.[45] Various combinations have been tried in the hope of reducing the bupivacaine concentration, to avoid unwanted muscle weakness and hypotension. However, none has been entirely satisfactory.

Infusions, to be effective, require a lot of adjustment and dermatome testing by the midwife.[46] In practice, it is difficult to achieve the proper balance between adequate analgesia and the risk of drug toxicity, hypotension and motor weakness. Inefficiently controlled infusions require regular top-ups by the anaesthetist. The addition of an opioid may improve the quality of pain relief particularly in the case of perineal pain or where there is a missed segment, but it does not avoid hypotension or forceps delivery. It also appears to be effective in abolishing shivering.[47] Analgesia may be improved somewhat in the first stage but is ineffective in the late first and second stage. Pruritis can be quite severe and troublesome to the mother.

Effectiveness of epidural opiates in post-operative pain relief

Pain relief is good and long-lasting and the mother is mobilised early. Many centres give one dose of epidural opiate and remove the catheter for reasons of reducing risk factors. The problems of subsequent pain relief, when it falls within the period during which no further systemic opiates should be administered, remain uncertain. A mother may be left in much pain during this period while senior anaesthetic advice is sought.

Urinary retention often presents the problem of catheterisation and discomfort. Pruritis continues to be a problem. In short, the risk/benefit ratio is too great.

Role of the nursing staff
Nursing staff have undertaken the responsibility for a form of analgesia about which they know very little. Formal training should be mandatory in the understanding of this form of analgesia, of the monitoring, recognition of complications and the treatment of side effects.

Twentieth century use of epidural opiates
There is an uneasy concern that we are not taking full precautions or that the precautions which we are taking are not scientifically based. Not many labour wards or obstetric hospitals have a high dependency unit so a compromise is made. The mother and baby together are sent back to the ward with a set of instructions to an already over-committed ward staff. Continuous monitoring of the patient is impossible because of the old-fashioned design of many hospitals; many patients are in two and four bedded rooms behind closed doors. Nurses stations are often remote from small wards. Respiratory observations are inadequate and usually limited to hourly respiratory rate. Instructions are given to nursing staff to avoid parenteral narcotics for a period which is nebulous. Naloxone is not adjacent to the patients, and queries exist as to whether it should be given intravenously or intramuscularly by nursing staff if necessary. The biggest failure is the lack of proper formal training of the nurses. Epidural opiates are frequently used in situations where there is no resident anaesthetist. Lack of finance and shortage of staff mean that we are unable to provide the facilities which should be mandatory for the proper care of mothers.

Sociological complications
There are many social and ethnic implications in the use of this form of analgesia. Many cultures do not have the same expectations of pain relief in labour and may feel cheated if deprived of the associated pain. Wealthy countries like America have pain management teams in which nurses and medical staff, including anaesthetists, are fully trained to manage all obstetric post-operative pain. They insist that naloxone and full resuscitative equipment is kept by the patient's bedside. The patients are well monitored and are seen regularly by the pain management team who are oncall over 24 hours. Third World countries and countries where the delivery rate is high have little time or money for such techniques.

Lack of properly conducted trials
A true assessment of the real situation is not possible because of the lack of evidence from properly conducted clinical trials. Large Scandinavian surveys, reporting the incidence of respiratory depression, are all retrospective and suffer from the usual pitfalls of

unreliable data. There is a need for a prospective survey, in which respiratory depression is clearly defined. This must be a study of sufficient size and well controlled so that we get a more realistic idea of this problem. To date, the use of epidural opiates has been by trial and error.

Conclusions

Obstetric anaesthetists are lulled into a false sense of security, dealing as they do with mostly young, fit women. But more and more problem cases are being reported. The ethical situation is ambiguous, and the medicolegal implications enormous. In the event of medical insurance being transferred to our health authorities, we may not in the future, because of more National Health Service constraints, have the same freedom of choice with potentially dangerous techniques. There is no conclusive evidence that epidural or intrathecal opiates provide analgesia which is superior to that produced by other routes, neither is there proof that there is improved morbidity or mortality in obstetrics with this technique. That respiratory depression occurs is undisputed. It occurs in an unpredictable manner. Safer and effective alternative analgesia exists and in the light of this, it could be argued that the use of epidural opiates today is tantamount to medical negligence.

* *

ARGUMENTS AGAINST: K. MacLeod

In 1848 Simpson wrote, 'The distress and pain which women often endure while they are struggling through a difficult labour are beyond description and seem to be more than human nature will be able to bear under any other circumstance'. The Bible too refers to the distress that can be caused by labour and delivery; typically, 'Wherefore do I see every man with his hands on his loins, as a woman in travail and all faces are turned into paleness'. (Jeremiah 30; 6). In this country, since Queen Victoria's time when religious objections were overcome by her actions, relief of pain in labour has been attempted in many different ways by many different practitioners with anaesthetists well to the fore. It therefore behoves us to continually seek out improved techniques for this purpose, evaluate them, make them as safe as possible and when there is an 'indication', use them for the benefit of the patient and her child.

In the 1989 volume of *Obstetric Anaesthesia Digest*, a journal that sets out to bring to the attention of obstetric anaesthetists throughout the world significant advances in obstetric anaesthesia by giving references to summaries of and comments on papers drawn from all reputable journals, there were 35 papers thought worthy of inclusion concerning the use of epidural or spinal opiates in obstetrics. In the 1988 volume of the same journal, there were 46 such papers presented for comment. In 1990, publication continues unabated.

In most centres in the United States of America where obstetric anaesthesia is practised in a specialised way, the use of epidural opiates and opiate/local anaesthetic mixtures is widespread. This in a country where claims for medical malpractice are an ever-present risk to even the most competent of practitioners. In the United Kingdom with, in comparison, less apparently fully trained personnel available on the 'shop floor', less assistance in the way of high dependency nursing and reduced numbers of appropriate monitoring devices, there are many centres which use epidural opiates quite routinely and with a negligible incidence of serious complications. It is with this background that epidural opiates in obstetrics practice should be considered.

What has been the reason for the rapid introduction of these techniques and are they safe? Should they be abandoned in obstetric anaesthetic practice as the motion under debate suggests?

Theoretical considerations

It had been suspected for many years that there existed endogenous substances that possessed opiate-like characteristics and were involved in control of pain in an unconscious way. Opioid receptors were first demonstrated in the brain in 1973[3] and in the spinal cord in 1976.[4] Analgesia was produced by spinally applied opiates in animals in the same year.[4] Three years later in 1979, Wang[7]*et al.* showed that in cancer patients, a subarachnoid injection of morphine produced long-lasting and profound analgesia and in the same year the use in man of epidural opiates was reported in *The Lancet*.[8]

It was not long before this new application of an established and well-known class of drugs through a well-known and readily available delivery system was being widely used throughout the developed world. Morgan listed the predicted advantages of spinally applied opiates which explain some of the enthusiasm for the technique:[49]

1.   Segmental analgesia with no sensory or motor loss;
2.   No autonomic block with consequent absence of hypotension;
3.   No central or respiratory depression;
4.   Availability of a large number of drugs;
5.   Existence of a specific antagonist.

The analgesic action of epidural and intrathecal opiates appears to be mediated by two distinct mechanisms: first, some systemic absorption which results in a central site of action in the conventional manner, and second, diffusion into the dorsal horn of the spinal cord via the cerebrospinal fluid and to the substantia gelatinosa. The small A delta and unmyelinated C fibres which conduct acute and slow pain respectively terminate at the substantia gelatinosa and it is here where opiates may bind with specific receptors to modulate pain transmission to the ascending anterolateral spinothalamic tracts (although some A delta fibres do bypass this region).

These potential advantages were not lost on obstetric anaesthetists and they soon were attempting to find applications for the technique.

Use of epidural opiates in obstetric anaesthesia

It soon became apparent that epidural application of opiates, although reducing the pain associated with labour, did not control it well enough in the latter part of the first stage and not at all in the second stage, even in high, approaching systemic, doses. Intrathecal administration was more effective but again relatively poor in the second stage and will not be considered further.

Justins[38] *et al.* studied this action of extradural fentanyl with bupivacaine to produce obstetric analgesia and compared the quality and duration of this analgesia with that produced by plain bupivacaine. Their results showed that this application indeed had a future.

The technique of combining local anaesthetics with fentanyl or other opiates is now widespread and many units, both in the UK and in the USA, advocate very low dose bupivacaine 0.125% or 0.0625% mixed with 50–100 μg fentanyl per 20 ml of solution and infusing this at a rate of 5–8 ml per hour. The advantages claimed are low incidence of motor block, reduced incidence and severity of sympathetic block and therefore hypotension and a (possible) reduction in instrumental deliveries.

The addition of an opiate to an existing local-anaesthetic-only epidural improves the quality of block in persistent missed segment and

Table 7.2 Synergistic mode of action of epidural local anaesthetic/opiate mix

LA	Afferent input to spinal cord via A delta and C fibres reduced
Opioid	Modulation of C and some A delta fibres at substantia gelatinosa. Reduced central transmission via spinothalamic tract

Table 7.3 Uses of epidural opiates in obstetric analgesia

1. Synergistic effect with local anaesthetic reduced dose less motor block
2. Reduces incidence of 'one-sided' and missed segment blocking
3. Alleviates persistent back and perineal pain
4. Reduced incidence and severity of 'shivering'
5. Less hypotension with less local anaesthetic
6. Post-operative delivery pain relief optimised

unilateral blocks, thereby reducing the need for large doses of local anaesthetic and/or resiting.

In labour where the head is failing to rotate and is posterior in position, occasionally local anaesthetics fail to relieve the back or perineal pain. Opiates, particularly fentanyl, are well known to be of great help in these situations.

Shivering can occasionally cause patients in labour a good deal of distress and there have been several studies to show that this trouble-some complication can be alleviated by the use of epidural opiates.[50,51]

In the patient who has congenital or acquired heart disease, major changes in sympathetic tone resulting in hypotension can have disas-trous consequences. Epidural opiates now have a major role to play in this area.[52,53]

The excellent analgesia particularly associated with the use of mor-phine and diamorphine after caesarean section has several advan-tages. Early mobilisation secondary to good pain relief will reduce the incidence of deep vein thrombosis. Painful, time-consuming and often inadequate intramuscular injections of opiates are avoided, thereby reducing the excretion into breast milk. Post-operative respiratory function, particularly in obese patients, will be improved and as a consequence, recovery will be optimised.

It is as well at this stage to define the properties of the ideal opiate required for epidural use in obstetrics. The ideal drug should exhibit the following characteristics:[54]

1. High lipid solubility;
2. High molecular weight;
3. Strong binding to receptor protein (prolonged effect);
4. Prolonged intrinsic activity;
5. No direct or indirect effect on the fetus.

We must now of course consider the complications and get some idea of the incidence of these and their severity in comparison with other pain relief techniques before we can consider the motion further.

Complications of epidural opiate and opiate local anaesthetic use

1. Pruritis;
2. Nausea and vomiting;
3. Urinary retention;
4. Sedation and/or mood change;
5. Unpredictable respiratory depression;
6. Herpes reactivation;
7. Complications associated with epidural catheterisation;
8. Complications of epidural local anaesthesia.

Of the above complications, seven are relatively uncommon or well known and can be dealt with easily. Because of its life-threatening nature, the eighth, unpredictable respiratory depression, is of more concern and will be discussed more fully.

Pruritis

Pruritis occurs in 40–70% of patients given epidural opiates and it seems that this incidence is the same for all the commonly available drugs, i.e. fentanyl, diamorphine, morphine and pethidine. Patients should be given the choice of whether they wish to go on with this form of pain relief or to abandon it in favour of another. About 10–15% will elect to take the alternative method. The symptoms can be reduced with antihistamines and abolished with naloxone but at the price of severely reduced analgesic efficiency. The pruritis will spontaneously resolve usually 3–4 hours after the last dose.

Nausea and vomiting

As can be seen from the list of intramuscular and intravenous opiate side effects below, nausea and vomiting are common to all methods of administration. Some series show a higher incidence in those patients given epidural opiates compared with those given the intramuscular form. Others give a similar incidence of about 30%. It appears that central brain stem opiate stimulation is the cause of the nausea and vomiting. Conventional anti-emetics help to reduce the symptoms but interestingly, naloxone appears to be of no value.

Urinary retention

This side effect is not related to intravenous or intramuscular use. Epidurally administered opiates will, shortly after their administration cause a marked relaxation of detrusor muscle function leading to an increase in bladder capacity and a marked tendency to urinary retention.[55] The effect is probably mediated by interference with sacral parasympathetic outflow and can be overcome by the use of naloxone which restores detrusor tone to normal.

The incidence is about 70% with reports varying from 57% to 80%.

Sedation and mood change

These effects are due to a central action whether by systemic absorption or cerebrospinal fluid circulation and though variable, can be expected to some degree in all patients.

Herpes reactivation

There has been some early work[56] suggesting a link between reactivation of genital herpes infection and the use of epidural opiates in the obstetric patient. Further studies will be required to establish the validity of this observation.

Complications associated with epidural catheterisation and epidural local anaesthetic administration are well known and will not be considered.

It is well to remember at this stage that other forms of opiate administration have their own specific as well as general drawbacks in use.

Side effects of IM opiate
administration
1. Poor analgesia
2. Nausea and vomiting
3. Central sedation
4. Repeated painful injections
5. Respiratory depression

Side effects of IV opiate
administration
1. Pruritis
2. Nausea and vomiting
3. Central sedation
4. Respiratory depression
5. Machine failure
6. Overdose

Respiratory depression

Respiratory depression is a complication common to all modes of opiate administration but obviously of great concern and potentially life-threatening if it is not recognised and treated. Respiratory depression has been extensively investigated in relation to epidural (and intrathecal) opiate use, many case reports have been published and series recorded. While the reported incidence of unpredictable respiratory depression varies from series to series, it has to be accepted that there is an incidence and precautions have to be taken to minimise and, as far as possible, remove all danger to the patient.

Factors predisposing to the development of respiratory depression in this clinical situation are said to be as follows:[16]

1. Advanced age;
2. Use of water soluble opioids;
3. Concomitant use of parenteral opioids;
4. Lack of tolerance to opioids;
5. Increased intrathoracic pressure;
6. Intrathecal administration;
7. Large doses;
8. Thoracic extradural opioids.

It is also well known that morphine, a relatively lipid insoluble drug, will be absorbed slowly across the dura into the CSF and then to its site of action. The drug remains in the CSF for a considerable length of time and has the potential for cephalad spread. A more logical choice, a fat soluble drug such as fentanyl, diamorphine or pethidine, will not have this propensity and these have been shown to have less of an incidence of respiratory depression.

Parenteral opiate administration can easily be avoided in obstetric patients. As most of them are young, there is rarely a lack of tolerance to opiates. Thoracic pressure is not raised. As already stated, intra-thecal use is not being considered. It goes without saying that large doses should be avoided and in obstetric anaesthetic practice (if not all), the thoracic epidural route is unnecessary.

Recommendations have also been made concerning where patients who have had epidural opiates need to be nursed:

1. Intensive care unit;
2. High dependency unit;
3. Stepdown or post-operative ward;
4. Ward;
5. Labour ward;

With the exception of the ordinary ward, all the other sites benefit from an increased level of nursing care, often on a one-to-one basis. They all will be able to offer a degree of monitoring appropriate to the level of staffing. The labour ward can really be considered as an intensive care situation.

Monitoring options that might be considered are as follows:

1. Respiratory inductance plethysmography;
2. Apnoea alarms;
3. Oximetry;
4. Capnography;
5. Transcutaneous CO_2 electrode;
6. Hourly respiratory count.

Of all these, the only practical solution for the obstetric patient is the hourly respiratory count, which will of course detect a falling rate. A bonus, of course, is that the individual doing the count will be able to observe the patient's general condition and a degree of unacceptable somnolence would be easily detected and attention quickly drawn to this state of affairs.

At St Mary's, the following instructions to the nursing staff are included in the notes for their guidance in dealing with these patients:

Epidural morphine/diamorphine
This patient has an epidural catheter in situ in order that epidural morphine can be administered for profound pain relief.

A.   All epidural opiate injections must be administered by a doctor as directed on the prescription sheet.

B.   No opiates should be administered by any other route during the time that epidural opiate analgesia is being used and for eight hours after the last epidural dose unless an anaesthetist is consulted.

C.   The respiratory rate must be recorded half-hourly for two hours and then hourly for six hours. If it falls below 10/minute contact an anaesthetist.

D.   Urinary output must be recorded until the epidural opiates are discontinued.

E.   Should 'itching' occur, an anaesthetist should be informed.

F.   If after 30 minutes the patient feels that pain has not been satisfactorily relieved or pain returns in less than four hours, an anaesthetist must be informed.

These guidelines, though far from comprehensive, have worked well for the past ten years since the relatively routine use of epidural opiates began in this hospital. The skills required by the nursing staff involved in the care of these patients are basically those of a State Registered Nurse. In the situations mentioned, particularly the labour ward, in addition to the basic nursing skills there are those of the midwife; a very experienced pair of hands!

Nursing skills required

1. O_2 administration (face mask);
2.   Bag and mask intermittent positive pressure ventilation;
3.   Naloxone IV/IM administration;
4.   Knowledge and availability of resuscitation trolley;
5.   Adequate staffing levels;
6.   Pain control instruction.

That these particular resuscitation skills have never been called into action speaks for itself. Indeed, there has been only one case report of respiratory depression associated with the use of epidural opiates in the obstetric patient in this country.[27] For a widely used technique to have so few reported serious side effects and yet to have been very effective could be regarded as a great strength.

The motion that is being debated in this paper is that epidural opiates should be abandoned in obstetric anaesthetic practice. Why so? To sum up, we have a relatively new application of a well-known family of drugs. The application seems to work well, better than conventional techniques, in a number of clinical situations. There are side effects, serious and not so serious, attached to all procedures carried out in medical practice and the risk-to-benefit ratio associated with each of these is the major determinant of their continuation. It is obvious that all forms of opiate administration have their potential problems. The **epidural** administration of opiates is no exception to this. These can be minimised in the interest of analgesic efficacy and safety for the patient in the manner outlined. Can we really deny our patients the benefits of good analgesia when we know that man is the master of the technique and not the technique the master of man?

There **is** a place for epidural opiates in obstetric anaesthetic practise. It must be used where indicated, it must be carefully controlled and in so doing the patient, her baby and her medical and midwifery attendants will benefit.

REFERENCES

1. Chakravarty T, Tucker W, Rosen M, Vickers MD. Comparison of buprenorphine and pethidine given on demand to relieve post-operative pain. *British Medical Journal* 1979; **2:** 895–7.
2. Tamsen A, Hartig P, Dahlstrom B, Lindstrom B, Hison Holmdahl M. Patient controlled analgesia therapy in the post-operative period. *Acta Anaesthesiologica Scandinavica* 1979; **23:** 462–70.
3. Pert CB, Snyder S. Opiate receptors: demonstration in nervous tissues. *Science* 1973; **179:** 1011.
4. Yaksh TL, Rudy TA. Analgesia mediated by a direct spinal action of narcotics. *Science* 1976; **192:** 1357.
5. Snyder SH. Opiate receptors and internal opiates. *Scientific American* 1977; **236:** 44–56.
6. Snyder SH. Opiate receptors in the brain. *New England Journal of Medicine* 1977; **296:** 266–71.
7. Wang JK, Nauss LE, Thomas JE. Pain relief by intrathecally applied morphine in man. *Anesthesiology* 1979; **50:** 149–51.
8. Behar M, Olshwang D, Magora F, Davidson JT. Epidural morphine in treatment of pain. *Lancet* 1979; **1:** 527–8.
9. Cousins MJ, Mather LE, Glynn CJ, Wilson PR, Graham JR. Selective spinal analgesia. *Lancet* 1979; **1:** 1141–2.
10. Nordberg G. Pharmacokinetic aspects of spinal morphine analgesia. *Acta Anaesthesiologica Scandinavica* 1984; **79**(Suppl 79): 1–38.
11. Cousins MJ, Bridenbaugh PO. Spinal opioids and pain relief in acute care. In: Cousins MJ, Philip GD (eds).
12. Way EL. Site and mechanisms of basic narcotic receptor function based on current research. *Ann Emerg Med* 1986; **15:** 1021–5.
13. Martin WR. Clinical evidence for different narcotic receptors and relevance for the clinician. *Ann Emerg Med* 1986; **15:** 1026–9.
14. Adams ML, Brase DA, Welch SP, Dewey WL. The role of endogenous peptides in the action of opioid analgesics. *Ann Emerg Med* 1986; **15:** 1030–5.
15. Sjostrand UH, Rawal N. Regional opioids in anaesthesiology and pain management. *Int Anaesthesiology Clinics* 1986; **24:** 2.
16. Cousins MJ, Mather LE. Intrathecal and epidural administration of opioids. *Anesthesiology* 1984; **61:** 276–310.

17. Martin R, Lamarche Y, Tetrault JP. Epidural and intrathecal narcotics. *Canadian Anaesthetists Society Journal* 1983; **30:** 662–73.
18. Kanto J, Erkkola R. Epidural and intrathecal opiates in obstetrics. *International Journal of Clinical Pharmacology* 1984; **22:** 316–23.
19. Scott DB, McClure J. Selective epidural analgesia. *Lancet* 1979; **2:** 356–7.
20. Glynn CJ, Mather LE, Cousins MJ, Wilson PR, Graham JR. Spinal narcotics and respiratory depression. *Lancet* 1979; **2:** 356–7.
21. Liolios A, Andersen FH. Selective spinal analgesia. *Lancet* 1979; **2:** 357.
22. Davies GK, Tolhurst-Cleaver CL, James TL. CNS depression from intrathecal morphine. *Anesthesiology* 1980; **52:** 280.
23. Davies GK, Tolhurst-Cleaver CL, James TL. Respiratory depression after intrathecal narcotics. *Anaesthesia* 1980; **35:** 1080–3.
24. Writer WDR, Hurtig JB, Edelist G, Evans D, Fox GS, Needs RE, Hope CE, Forrest JB. Epidural morphine prophylaxis of post-operative pain: report of a double-blind multicentre study. *Canadian Anaesthetists Society Journal* 1985; **32:** 330–8.
25. Davies GK, Tolhurst-Cleaver CL, James TL. Respiratory depression after intrathecal narcotics. *Anaesthesia* 1981; **36:** 268–76.
26. Wust HJ, Bromage PR. Delayed respiratory arrest after epidural hydromorphone. *Anaesthesia* 1987; **42:** 404–6.
27. Brockway MS. Profound respiratory depression after extraduval feutany. *British Journal of Anaesthesia* 1990; **64:** 243–5.
28. McCaughey W, Graham JL. The respiratory depression of epidural morphine: time course and effect of posture. *Anaesthesia* 1982; **37:** 990–5.
29. Rawal N, Armer S, Gustafsson LL, Allvin R. Present state of extradural and intrathecal opioid analgesia in Sweden. *British Journal of Anaesthesia* 1987; **59:** 791–9.
30. Mehnert JH, Dupont TJ, Rose DH. Intermittent epidural morphine instillation for control of post-operative pain. *Canadian Anaesthetists Society Journal* 1986; **33:** 542–9.
31. Abboud TK, Moore M, Zhu J *et al*. Epidural butorphanol or morphine for the relief of post-caesarean section pain: ventilatory responses to carbon dioxide. *Anesthesia and Analgesia* 1987; **66:** 887–93.
32. Kotelko DM, Dailey P, Schnider SM, Rosen MA, Hughes SC, Brizgys RV. Epidural morphine analgesia after caesarean delivery. *Obstetrics and Gynecology* 1984; **63:** 409–13.
33. Leicht CH, Hughes SC, Dailey PA, Schnider SM, Rosen MA. Epidural morphine sulfate for analgesia after caesarean section: a prospective report of 1000 patients. *Anesthesiology* 1986; **65:** A366.
34. McMorland GH, Douglas JD. Epidural morphine for post-operative analgesia. *Canadian Anaesthetists Society Journal* 1986; **33:** 115–6.
35. Skjoldbrand A, Garle M, Gustafsson LL, Johansson H, Lunnell N-O, Rane A. Extradural pethidine with and without adrenaline during labour: wide variation in effect. *British Journal of Anaesthesia* 1982; **54:** 415–20.
36. Husemeyer RP, Cummings AJ, Rosankiewicz JR, Davenport HT. A study of pethidine kinetics and analgesia in women during labour fol-

lowing intravenous, intramuscular and epidural administration. *British Journal of Clinical Pharmacology* 1982; **13:** 171–6.

37. Naulty JS, Malinow A, Hunt CO, Hausheer J, Datta S, Lema MJ, Ostheimer GW. Epidural butorphanol-bupivacaine for analgesia during labour and delivery. *Anesthesiology* 1986; **65:** A396.

38. Justins D, Francis DM, Houlton PG, Reynolds F. A controlled trial of extradural fentanyl in labour. *British Journal of Anaesthesia* 1982; **54:** 409–14.

39. Justins DM, Knott C, Luthman J, Reynolds F. Epidural versus intramuscular fentanyl: analgesia and pharmacokinetics in labour. *Anaesthesia* 1983; **38:** 937–42.

40. Vella LM, Willatts DG, Knott C, Lintin DJ, Justins DM, Reynolds F. Epidural fentanyl in labour: an evaluation of the systemic contribution to anaesthesia. *Anaesthesia* 1985; **40:** 741–7.

41. Cohen SE, Tan S, Albright GA, Halpern J. Epidural fentanyl/bupivacaine for obstetric analgesia. *Anesthesiology* 1987; **67:** 403–7.

42. Van Steenberge A, Debroux HC, Noorduin H. Extradural bupivacaine with sufentanil for vaginal delivery: a double-blind trial. *British Journal of Anaesthesia* 1987; **59:** 1518–22.

43. Phillips GH. Epidural sufentanil/bupivacaine combinations for analgesia during labour: effect of varying sufentanil dose. *Anesthesiology* 1987; **67:** 835–8.

44. Little MS, McNitt JD, Choi HJ, Tremper KK. A pilot study of low dose epidural sufentanil and bupivacaine for labour analgesia. *Anesthesiology* 1987; **67:** A444.

45. Reynolds F, O'Sullivan G. Epidural fentanyl and perineal pain in labour. *Anaesthesia* 1989; **44:** 341–4.

46. Gaylord DG, Wilson IH, Balmer HGR. An epidural infusion technique for labour. *Anaesthesia* 1987; **42:** 1098–1101.

47. Johnson MD, Sevarino FB, Lema MJ, Datta S, Ostheimer GW, Naulty JS. Effect of epidural sufentanil on temperature regulation in the parturient. *Anesthesiology* 1987; **67:** A450.

48. Johnson MD, Sevarino FB, Lema MJ. Cessation of shivering and hypothermia associated with epidural sufentanil. *Anesthesia and Analgesia* 1989; **68:** 70–71.

49. Morgan M. The rational use of intrathecal and extradural opiates. *British Journal of Anaesthesia* 1989; **63:** 165–88.

50. Casey WF *et al.* Intravenous meperidine (pethidine) for control of shivering during caesarean section under epidural anaesthesia. *Canadian Journal of Anaesthesia* 1988; **35:** 128–33.

51. Sevarioin FB. The effect of epidural sufentanil on shivering and body temperature in the parturient. *Anesthesia and Analgesia* 1989; **68:** 530–3.

52. Robinson DE, Leicht CH. Epidural analgesia with low dose bupivacaine and fentanyl for labour and delivery in a parturient with severe pulmonary hypertension. *Anesthesiology* 1988; **68:** 285–8.

53. Power KJ, Avery AF. Extradural analgesia in the intrapartum management of a parturient with pulmonary hypertension. *British Journal of Anaesthesia* 1989; **63:** 116–20.

54. Bilsback P *et al.* Efficiency of epidural administration of lofentanyl,

bupremorphine or saline in the management of post-operative pain. *British Journal of Anaesthesia* 1985; **57**: 943.

55. Rawal N *et al*. An experimental study of urodynamic effects of epidural morphine and of naloxone reversal. *Anesthesia and Analgesia* 1983; **62**: 641.

56. Crone L *et al*. Recurrent herpes simplex virus labialis and the use of epidural morphine in obstetric patients. *Anesthesia and Analgesia* 1988; **67**: 318–23.

8

Spinal anaesthesia for caesarean section must only be performed in the presence of a consultant anaesthetist

ARGUMENTS FOR: D. Brighouse

Spinal anaesthesia has enjoyed a considerable revival during the 1980s, particularly in obstetric practice. The major contra-indications to spinal and epidural anaesthesia are essentially the same: namely, coagulation abnormalities and actual or anticipated hypovolaemia. Patients falling into these groups will require general anaesthetics. For all other mothers wishing to remain awake for caesarean section, the choice lies between spinal and epidural anaesthesia.

Devotees of spinal anaesthesia claim that the technique is superior to epidural anaesthesia for several reasons:

1. Speed of insertion;
2. Speed of onset of the block;
3. No drug toxicity;
4. Quality of analgesia.

Spinal anaesthesia also has a number of disadvantages, namely:

1. Hypotension;
2. Motor block;
3. Headache;
4. Discontinuous technique.

These advantages and disadvantages will now be discussed.

Speed of insertion
The insertion of a spinal needle is theoretically a simpler procedure than the insertion of an epidural needle and catheter, and should therefore be quicker. This is probably true with larger (e.g. 22 g) spinal needles, but the very fine spinal needles currently in use in

obstetric practice may be difficult to insert. A failure rate of 8% has been reported following attempted lumbar puncture with 29 g needles.[1]

The speed of insertion of spinal versus epidural is not of major clinical relevance. The mother without analgesia requiring caesarean section for severe fetal distress will continue to need a general anaesthetic.

Speed of onset

The rate of onset of surgical anaesthesia following intrathecal injection of local anaesthetic is usually faster than after extradural injection. However, this depends on the type of local anaesthetic and on the way in which the mother is positioned. A study using 1% tetracaine in 10% dextrose in identical volumes showed that sensory anaesthesia to T4 developed within five minutes when lumbar puncture in the right lateral position was followed by turning to the left wedged position, but that lumbar puncture in the left lateral position followed by the left wedged position resulted in failure to achieve adequate anaesthesia for caesarean section.[2]

Another study using intrathecal isobaric 0.5% bupivacaine for caesarean section showed an extension of anaesthetic level of up to seven segments associated with turning from the lateral to supine wedged position.[3]

A study of 30 patients undergoing elective caesarean section with intrathecal hyperbaric 5% lignocaine demonstrated that all but one patient achieved a block suitable for surgery within nine minutes of intrathecal injection. However, in four of the patients the block continued to extend after nine minutes, reaching a final height of C2. These four patients all complained of inability to breathe, and all four had dysphagia.[4]

The differing results of these studies suggest that careful positioning of the patient undergoing spinal anaesthesia for caesarean section is vital if the technique is to remain safe. This positioning involves using pillows or wedges to reproduce the cervical and thoracic spinal curvature whilst the patient is in the lateral position, and thus stop the local anaesthetic solution running 'uphill' into the cervical nerve roots (Carrie, personal communication). Whilst effective in maintaining the safety of the technique, this increases the time taken to achieve surgical anaesthesia to about 20 minutes.

The use of extradural pH-adjusted 0.5% bupivacaine with adrenaline provides surgical anaesthesia in 20–40 minutes,[5] and pH-adjusted extradural 2% lignocaine with adrenaline provides sensory blockade to T5 at ten minutes.[6]

It therefore appears that by selection of suitable local anaesthetic solutions for extradural use, the speed of onset of surgical anaesthesia differs only marginally between spinal and epidural techniques. Certainly this difference is rarely likely to be of clinical importance.

Drug toxicity
This is one of the few undeniable advantages of spinal compared with epidural anaesthesia. A very small mass of drug produces a profound effect; thus there is never a risk of approaching toxic concentrations of local anaesthetic.

Quality of analgesia
Spinal anaesthesia undoubtedly produces a dense block. In addition to the sympathetic block and loss of temperature and pain sensation, there is also almost complete blockade of deep pressure, somatic motor and proprioceptive fibres. This degree of anaesthesia does not occur with epidural injection. Nevertheless a recent study comparing the incidence of visceral pain during caesarean section under spinal or epidural anaesthesia showed no difference between the two groups.[7]

Although at first sight the more profound spinal analgesia would appear desirable, in practice many mothers particularly dislike the prolonged motor block and loss of proprioceptive sense which occurs. A number of mothers having repeat caesarean section under epidural anaesthesia after previous sections under spinal block have spontaneously voiced their preference for the epidural technique (personal observation).

Hypotension
Any fall in maternal blood pressure will be accompanied by reduction in uteroplacental blood flow, thus compromising fetal well-being. Further falls in maternal blood pressure will, of course, jeopardise maternal safety.

All women undergoing caesarean section are at particular risk of aortocaval compression, because they are unable to assume the full lateral position on the operating table. A regional block which causes paralysis of the efferent vasomotor fibres will compound any hypotension. Hypotension occurs more frequently and more rapidly with spinal rather than epidural block due to the speed of onset and density of the block. Some authors have quoted an incidence of hypotension as high as 64% during spinal analgesia for caesarean section.[3]

In order to prevent hypotension occurring with spinal anaesthesia, many experts advocate the use of prophylactic ephedrine. This may well prevent hypotension, but if large doses of ephedrine are used this may in itself be detrimental to fetal well-being. A recent study showed a significant increase in acidosis (measured in cord blood at delivery) in babies born by elective caesarean section under spinal anaesthesia compared with epidural.[8]

Motor block

Maternal dislike of prolonged motor block has already been discussed. However the profound motor block resulting from spinal anaesthesia also has significant implications for maternal safety. The well-nourished pregnant mother at term may weigh 70–80 kg, and sometimes considerably more. Under the influence of spinal anaesthesia the mother is unable to move herself at all. Moving such a 'dead weight' into the full lateral position during initiation of anaesthesia may be a physical impossibility for a small anaesthetist with a single assistant, but assumption of such a position may, on occasion, be life-saving. During epidural anaesthesia not only is rapid onset of hypotension less common, but motor block is usually less complete.

Headache

Post-dural puncture headache (PDPH) is well described,[9] and it is known that pregnant women are at particularly high risk.[10] In an effort to minimise this complication, junior anaesthetists are taught to insert spinal needles with the bevel parallel to the longitudinal axis of the spinal cord, and to use the smallest size of spinal needle available. Despite these precautions, a recent study of over 2500 women receiving spinal anaesthesia for caesarean section demonstrated a PDPH rate of 5–10%. Dural puncture had been performed by experienced residents under direct supervision, or by attending anaesthetists themselves, using 26 g needles.[11] This headache rate is higher than the expected rate of inadvertent dural tap occurring with epidural insertion in a teaching unit.[12] In one series of 964 caesarean sections performed under epidural block, the incidence of inadvertent dural tap was zero.[13]

Post-dural puncture headache will, therefore, remain an unpredictable sequel to spinal rather than epidural anaesthesia, and cannot be regarded as a minor complication. The need to remain bedbound and supine for the first few days after delivery is not only distressing for the mother but also reduces the chances of successfully establishing breastfeeding.

Discontinuous technique

One of the major limitations of spinal anaesthesia is the inflexibility of the technique. There is no provision for supplementing intra-operative analgesia, or for giving post-operative analgesia. Attempts to overcome these problems have followed two routes:

a)   continuous spinal analgesia via intrathecal catheters;
b)   combined epidural and spinal block.

Use of intrathecal catheters has, so far, proved disappointing. 'Micro' catheters (30 or 32 gauge) introduced through fine spinal needles have failed to add versatility to spinal techniques because of technical difficulties with their use.

Combined epidural and spinal block is, therefore, the only available method of augmenting the 'single shot' spinal. Both needle-through-needle[14] and separate epidural and spinal injection[15] have been described. Although effective in improving the versatility of spinal blockade alone, the need for combined techniques is surely proof of the limitations of spinal anaesthesia for caesarean section.

Summary
The arguments for the use of spinal rather than epidural analgesia for caesarean section have been discussed. It is the author's opinion that the perceived benefits of spinal anaesthesia are very much outweighed by its limitations, unless augmented by epidural block. Moreover, for the unsupervised junior anaesthetist, the risk of rapidly occurring severe hypotension will remain a major danger of spinal anaesthesia for caesarean section.

*   *

ARGUMENTS AGAINST: J. Clarke

My major objection to the proposal is that it is not, in my view, based either on clinical experience or common sense. To my knowledge there is no data to suggest that spinals in the hands of non-consultants are unsafe, so where does such a notion come from? I can only presume from consultants trying out spinals and finding an extremely rapid sequence of physiological changes which, I freely admit, I found worrying when I first started using spinals for caesarean section. However, the learning curve is reassuringly steep, and meetings such as this permit 'tricks of the trade' to be rapidly disseminated, so that we do not all have to cover the same ground repeatedly.

My second objection is that all the side effects of spinals can occur whilst carrying out epidurals, usually without the benefit of forward planning and using doses of local anaesthetic that far exceed those used for spinals, resulting in potentially much greater changes in the patient's physiological status. Is it not standard teaching that all the effects are correctable? Does this then mean that only consultants should carry out epidurals?

My third objection is that the concept of 'Consultants Only' exists nowhere else in anaesthesia, so why spinals for caesarean section? If such a concept should ever occur, there are many more deserving cases such as neonatal anaesthesia, management of the difficult airway, care of the ITU patient, deliberate hypotension, to name but a few on a very long list before spinals would appear.

Spinals are technically easy to perform, most SHOs are competent within a few months of starting anaesthesia of carrying them out for emergency hip surgery, urology, etc. Furthermore, though there is an exaggerated physiological response to spinals in the obstetric patient, these are predictable and manoeuvres to limit them are well known, as are the necessary treatments. This is the reason that they have found such favour in Third World obstetric patients.

Lastly, in my view, one of the major attractions of spinals is that they permits a rapid caesarean section to be carried out. Until recently in this country, a mother needing an urgent section was often only offered a general anaesthetic, since epidurals can take too long. This has denied many couples the pleasure of an awake casearean section. Now we have a method almost as rapid as general anaesthesia. Furthermore most emergency sections are carried out by junior staff and the hazards of misplaced endotracheal tubes, aspiration and awareness are known to us all. Is it not better to teach a technique that preserves consciousness, thus permitting continuous monitoring of the patient's cerebral status?

I strongly believe in a consultant-led anaesthetic service but surely we are capable of training our junior staff to the standard necessary to carry out spinal anaesthesia for caesarean section for, if not, how can we claim we are training the next generation of consultant anaesthetists?

REFERENCES

1. Flaatten H, Rodt SA, Vamnes J *et al.* Postdural puncture headache: a comparison between 26 and 29 gauge needles in young patients. *Anaesthesia* 1989; **44:** 147–9.
2. Sprague DH. Effects of position and uterine displacement on spinal anesthesia for cesarean section. *Anesthesiology* 1976; **44:** 164–6.
3. Russell IF. Spinal anaesthesia for caesarean section: the use of 0.5% bupivacaine. *British Journal of Anaesthesia* 1983; **55:** 309–14.
4. Bembridge M, Macdonald R, Lyons G. Spinal anaesthesia with hyperbaric lignocaine for elective caesarean section. *Anaesthesia* 1986; **41:** 906–9.
5. Tackley RM, Coe AJ. Alkalinised bupivacaine and adrenaline for epidural caesarean section: a comparison with 0.5% bupivacaine. *Anaesthesia* 1988; **43:** 1019–21.
6. Di Fazio CA, Carron H, Grosslight KR *et al.* Comparison of pH-adjusted solutions for epidural lidocaine anaesthesia. *Anesthesia and Analgesia* 1986; **66:** 791–4.
7. Alahuhta S, Kangas-Saarela T, Hollmen AI, Edstrom HH. Visceral

pain during caesarean section under spinal and epidural anaesthesia with bupivacaine. *Acta Anaesthesia Scand* 1990; **34:** 95–8.

8. Ratcliffe FM. Neonatal acid-base status after general, spinal or extradural anaesthesia for caesarean section. *British Journal of Anaesthesia* 1990; **64:** 381P–82P.

9. Bonica JJ. *Principles and practice of obstetric analgesia and anesthesia.* Philadelphia: FA Davis, 1972.

10. Vandam LD. Neurologic sequelae of spinal and epidural anaesthesia. *Int Anesthesiol Clin* 1986; **24:** 231–55.

11. Naulty JS, Hertwig L, Hunt CO *et al.* Influence of local anesthetic solution on postdural puncture headache. *Anesthesiology* 1990; **72:** 450–4.

12. Holdcroft A, Morgan M. Maternal complications of obstetric epidural analgesia. *Anaesthesia and Intensive Care* 1976; **4:** 108–12.

13. Crawford JS, Davies P, Lewis M. Some aspects of epidural block provided for elective caesarean section. *Anaesthesia* 1984; **41:** 1039–46.

14. Carrie LES, O'Sullivan GM. Subarachnoid bupivacaine 0.5% for caesarean, section. *European Journal of Anaesthesiology* 1984; **1:** 275–83.

15. Brownridge P. Epidural and subarachnoid analgesia for elective caesarean section. *Anaesthesia* 1981; **36:** 70.

9

Update on some earlier controversies

D. Browne and H. Powell

Obstetrical anaesthetics is a super-specialty, a subgroup of a subgroup. It poses challenges commensurate with its unique contribution to human birth. Within this intense arena the anaesthetist, when confronted by a fence, is denied the comfort of sitting on it. There is compulsion not only to take a side but also to engage vigorously in its defence. In this feverish milieu, *Controversies in Obstetric Anaesthesia* was first published in 1990. This chapter reviews some of the subjects discussed then and the body of evidence which has accumulated since then.

It will come as no surprise to summarise that none of the controversies in Volume I has been resolved. We have fleshed out the bones of contention, but the skeleton remains. That is science.

Antacid prophylaxis in obstetrics
Since the Controversies debates covering the use of antacids during labour, there have been a number of papers in the journals relating to this topic. These include two reviews of current practice: one in the UK and one in Australia, and articles on famotidine, omeprazole, the effect of H_2 antagonists on plasma local anaesthetic levels and critical gastric volume and pulmonary aspiration.

Reviews of current practice

The recent review of antacid prophylaxis in the UK[1] carried out in November 1988 revealed that the most frequently used antacid prophylaxis is now a combination of ranitidine and sodium citrate for both elective and emergency caesarean section (LSCS). There is continuing controversy about the use of prophylaxis for all women in active labour and in most cases it is reserved for those patients at high risk for LSCS or instrumental delivery. Oral ranitidine 6-hourly is the regimen of choice. The Australian study[2] was carried out in 1987 and the results differed considerably from those in the British study. There was a lower incidence of prophylaxis for elective LSCS and a much higher use of particulate antacid compounds. Particulate antacids were still used for prophylaxis during labour in a number of hospitals and either particulate antacid or sodium citrate was the agent of choice for emergency LSCS. Use of H_2 antagonists was uncommon in all groups: <4% emergency and <12% elective LSCS.

A combination of effervescent cimetidine and sodium citrate has been evaluated for prophylaxis in both elective and emergency LSCS and although the combination was more effective than sodium citrate alone, it did not produce pH >2.5 in all patients.[3]

Brock-Utne and colleagues investigated the effect of ranitidine 50 mg intravenously (IV) pre-operatively in emergency LSCS together with 30 ml sodium citrate, metoclopramide and a vagolytic agent pre-induction. They found that no patient was at risk of low pH using this regimen.[4]

Sodium bicarbonate ($NaHCO_3$ 8.4%) as a single 20 ml oral bolus does not provide adequate antacid prophylaxis before LSCS[5] but may be used as an alternative to sodium citrate pre-induction in combination with 6-hourly oral ranitidine.

Famotidine

A new, potent, highly specific competitive H_2 antagonist called famotidine is now in clinical use and currently undergoing investigation in obstetric patients, although there are no published results as yet. When given as a single oral dose on the evening before surgery in non-obstetric patients, the effects on gastric volume and pH were very similar to those obtained with ranitidine.[6] Given as a single oral dose two hours before surgery,[7] there was no significant difference between famotidine and ranitidine with respect to pH. Famotidine significantly reduced gastric volume compared with ranitidine although no patient had a gastric aspirate greater than 25 ml. A parenteral preparation of famotidine also exists but is not licensed for clinical use in this country. A study using IV famotidine or ranitidine before surgery in morbidly obese patients found famotidine and ranitidine to be similarly effective in reducing gastric volume and pH but not always successful in bringing gastric volume and pH out of the risk categories for acid aspiration.[8]

Omeprazole

Omeprazole is a substituted benzimidazole derivative which inhibits gastric acid secretion by a unique new mechanism of action. It blocks the activity of the enzyme responsible for the gastric proton pump, effectively inhibiting gastric acid secretion regardless of the nature of the stimulus. It is now available as an oral preparation for general clinical use and there is an IV preparation currently undergoing phase II clinical trials. Investigating the effect of a single oral dose of 80 mg omeprazole on the evening before elective LSCS, Moore et al.[9] found that this regimen did not reliably produce gastric pH >2.5 and volume <25 ml in all patients. However, Gin et al.[10] found that omeprazole 40 mg orally on the evening before and the morning of surgery did produce gastric pH >2.5 and volume <25 ml in all patients. Ewart and colleagues[11] found this regimen superior to ranitidine for elective LSCS but further studies are required to assess the value of this agent before emergency LSCS. A single 40 mg IV dose one or three hours pre-operatively in general surgery patients did not always produce pH >3.5.[12]

H_2 antagonists and local anaesthetic plasma levels

Now that H_2 antagonist prophylaxis has become an accepted practice before LSCS, there has been some anxiety as to whether this might affect plasma levels of local anaesthetic agents during epidural blockade. A number of studies have investigated the effect of cimetidine and ranitidine on plasma concentrations of lignocaine and bupivacaine following single doses of the H_2 antagonists.[13-16] However, only one group has looked at patients given H_2 antagonists administered in the usual way, i.e. oral H_2 antagonist on the evening before and the morning of the operation, and they found no significant effect on bupivacaine clearance.[17]

Kishikawa et al. have investigated plasma lignocaine levels in patients undergoing major general surgical procedures with epidural and found that plasma lignocaine levels were significantly higher in the group treated with cimetidine compared with those given famotidine or placebo.[18]

Critical gastric volume and pulmonary aspiration

Recent studies in animals suggest that the critical volume of gastric aspirate required to produce aspiration pneumonitis may be greater than the 25 ml previously suggested. Raidoo et al. instilled human gastric aspirate (pH1, volume 0.4 ml/kg) into the tracheas of monkeys and found no clinical signs of aspiration pneumonitis.[19] More recently, they found that instillation of gastric content of pH1, 0.4 ml/kg in juvenile monkeys produced mild to moderate clinical and radiological changes, and volume >0.8 ml/kg produced increasingly severe pneumonitis with 50% mortality at 1 ml/kg. Extrapolated to humans, this would suggest a critical volume nearer to 50 ml (0.8 ml/kg) rather than the 25 ml usually quoted.[20]

Management of fulminating PET belongs in the hands of the anaesthetist

Since the Controversies debate on management of PET, there has been a considerable amount in the literature relating to the management of patients with this condition. Brown[21] suggests that it should be based upon discussion between the obstetrician, neonatologist, physician/intensivist and anaesthetist, and Mudie and Lewis[22] stress the necessity for pooled knowledge and teamwork.

Monitoring

Monitoring of these patients is a very controversial issue. At present most patients requiring central venous pressure (CVP) monitoring can be managed in an obstetric unit. However, management of a pulmonary artery catheter or direct arterial pressure monitoring would require admission to the intensive care unit (ICU). Van Assche[23] proposed that these patients should be admitted to a high-risk pregnancy unit before, during and after delivery. This unit would be situated close to the labour suite with permanent supervision by obstetric and anaesthetic staff. Similarly Duncan[24] states that, wherever possible, the treatment of sick patients with severe PET should take place only where high dependency care can be provided with invasive monitoring if required. Most obstetric units in the UK do not have this facility and doctors have to choose between managing these patients in the labour ward or in the ICU. In a retrospective study reviewing obstetric admissions to the ICU in Nottingham over a five year period, Graham[25] noted that 56% of obstetric admissions to the ICU (13 patients) were for PET, and of those patients, two died. Twelve patients had CVP monitoring and three had a pulmonary artery catheter.

Several papers argue the pros and cons of CVP versus PCWP monitoring in patients with complications related to central volume status, e.g. pulmonary oedema, persistent oliguria and intractable severe hypertension. Many state that CVP is not an accurate index of left heart filling pressure in these patients[21,23,26–30] but others suggest that CVP is a useful guide if it is low but unreliable if greater than 6–8 mmHg.[24,31] Some suggest that PCWP is no more useful than CVP.[32]

Measurement of PCWP, cardiac index (CI) and systemic vascular resistance (SVR) allows the most appropriate management of these patients who may require increased intravascular volume, fluid restriction or afterload or pre-load reduction.[33] Although in most cases it is possible to manage these patients without invasive monitoring by assuming that the patient is hypovolaemic with a high SVR and good myocardial function, the occasional patient who does not fit this category may be severely compromised. Without invasive monitoring it is not possible to predict which treatment regimen is appropriate in any individual patient.[29]

Convulsions

Controversy continues concerning the management of eclamptic fitting, both for prophylactic and acute treatment. For prevention, some advocate phenytoin[32,34,35b] while others support magnesium sulphate[23,35a,36,37] although both are also criticised.[34,35b,38] Intravenous diazepam[21,32,35b] or magnesium sulphate[35a,37] are recommended for the acute management of eclamptic fitting. There has also been a case report describing the successful use of clonazepam in controlling generalised myoclonic convulsions without sedation.[39]

Blood pressure management

Control of arterial blood pressure is the most important treatment to avoid the cerebral complications of PET.

Although control of acute hypertension is necessary to prevent intracerebral haemorrhage, brain damage in eclamptic patients can also be caused by cerebral ischaemia and hypoxia. Patients with eclampsia frequently have cerebral oedema and raised intracranial pressure. When arterial blood pressure is reduced too quickly and to a level lower than that necessary to maintain cerebral perfusion in the face of raised ICP, cerebral ischaemia and hypoxia can worsen. Close monitoring of arterial blood pressure is very important during antihypertensive and anticonvulsant therapy.[23]

Since severe hypertension of pregnancy may be associated with a relative increase in thromboxane A2 in relation to prostacyclin (PGI2), it has been suggested[23] that a therapeutic approach with a thromboxane synthetase inhibitor in combination with a thromboxane receptor blocker merits further investigation. This technique would act locally in damaged zones of vasculopathy without the adverse and generalised effects of potent antihypertensive treatment.

Hydralazine remains the most popular drug for reducing arterial blood pressure in pre-eclamptic patients, although its use has been implicated in worsening capillary leak and oedema.[32] Urapadil has also been used recently with good results: it reduces blood pressure by reducing SVR without increasing ICP[33] Angiotensin converting enzyme (ACE) inhibitors and prostacyclin are contra-indicated as they may cause poor fetal outcome.[21,32,40] Sodium nitroprusside is the best acute hypotensive agent for serious, resistant or complicated hypertension, when accompanied by a plasma infusion to overcome severe hypovolaemia. However, administration should be monitored by direct arterial pressure measurement and limited to a maximum of six hours to avoid the risk of cyanide toxicity in the fetus.[32] Glyceryl trinitrate (GTN) is well suited to use in patients with PET complicated by pulmonary oedema. Its use is not advisable in uncomplicated PET without prior volume resuscitation.[40] Intravenous labetalol may also be used,[22,32,36,40] nifedipine[21,32,40,41] diazoxide[23,40,41] or magnesium sulphate.[32] Droperidol may be useful as a combined sympatholytic and sedative agent for preventing sympathetic surges associated with agitation.[32]

Fluid management

Recommendations relating to fluid management in these patients vary. Hernandez *et al.*[36] stated that they keep their patients fluid restricted with fluid intake 100 ml/hr Hartmanns solution! They state that empirical use of diuretics should be avoided unless there is pulmonary oedema, although Baker[32] advocates use of an osmotic diuretic, e.g. mannitol, to encourage diuresis to prevent renal damage. Wasserstrum *et al.*[42] gave rapid infusions of 5% albumin solution 500 ml or 1000 ml to patients with PCWP <12 mmHg and found that it caused an increase in PCWP and CI, a decrease in SVR, an unchanged systemic MAP but significantly increased pulmonary MAP. They do not recommend such rapid infusion for routine clinical care. Most advocate use of human albumin solution for intravascular volume expansion provided there is no oedema. In patients with significant oedema there is likely to be increased capillary permeability with high risk of non-cardiogenic pulmonary oedema and cerebral oedema if volume overloaded. It is suggested that patients with oedema, oliguria and renal insufficiency need to be managed in an intensive care setting with fluid management guided by PCWP measurement.[21]Kirshon *et al.* gave 25% albumin to hypertensive, proteinuric patients with full invasive monitoring to increase the colloid osmotic pressure (COP) above 17 mmHg and then 5% albumin to increase the PCWP over 10 mmHg. If at any time the PCWP increased to greater than 15 mmHg, they were given 10–20 mg frusemide. MAP was controlled using sodium nitroprusside, glyceryl trinitrate or hydralazine. Using this regimen, no patient developed pulmonary oedema.[28]

Kirshon and colleagues have also investigated the value of dopamine in hypertensive, proteinuric, oliguric patients. The PCWP was increased to over 8 mmHg and then dopamine 1–5 µg/kg/min administered to maintain urine output greater than 0.5 ml/kg/hr. Dopamine at low dose selectively dilates renal vessels and increases renal blood flow, glomerular filtration rate and sodium excretion. In this study, following low dose dopamine there was an increase in urine output and cardiac output, decreased SVR and unchanged systemic arterial pressure.[33]

The pathogenesis of PET appears to involve a true or relative deficiency state of vasodepressor, anti-platelet-aggregator prostaglandins.[43] A possible treatment option might be by replacement to compensate for the prostaglandin deficiency. The E series of prostaglandins (PGs) are unsuitable as they have a high ratio of uterine stimulation to vasodepressor properties. However, the A series produce weak uterine stimulation but have strong hypotensive effects, probably by direct peripheral arteriolar dilation. In addition, work to date suggests that treatment with PGA1 could markedly improve renal function. Toppozada *et al.*[43] evaluated the use of PGA1 for induction of labour in patients with PET with an unripe cervix. Labour was successfully induced, blood pressure was reduced and maintained at normal levels and renal function improved.

The anaesthetist's contribution to the care of fulminating preeclamptic patients is summarised in the 1985–87 *Confidential Equiries into Maternal Death in the UK*. Anaesthetic staff should be involved early in the management of women with severe pre-eclampsia, even if operative delivery is not planned, to assist with analgesia, sedation, antihypertensive therapy and monitoring.[44]

Epidural controversies reviewed
- Midwife top-ups must be abandoned
- Withholding top-ups in the second stage is barbaric
- Primiparae can be reassured that epidural analgesia does not increase the incidence of forceps delivery

Midwife top-ups must be abandoned
Papers relating to the topic of midwife epidural top-ups include references to test doses, infusions and patient-controlled epidural analgesia (PCEA).

Test dose

There have been suggestions that a test dose should be given before each epidural top-up. However a test dose cannot reliably detect intravenous injection[45,46,47,48,49] and although many different regimens have been recommended for detecting inadvertent subarachnoid injection,[45,48,49,50] there is no clear test drug available.[48] If hyperbaric preparations are used then this produces extra work and an extra source of error as two drugs have to be checked and then administered. Also a midwife is unable to assess whether the block that results from a test dose is epidural or subarachnoid.[51]

An alternative test is the aspiration test but this may produce false negative results and to improve accuracy, the bacterial filter should be removed.[52]

Multihole catheters produce a potential problem with top-ups as, if placed partly within the epidural space and partly subdural or subarachnoid, a slow injection may deposit the local anaesthetic predominantly in the epidural space, but a fast injection may deposit a significant volume of the local anaesthetic in the subdural or subarachnoid space.[51] Epidural injections should always be given slowly and in small incremental doses of less than 5 ml. If low concentration solutions are used this should virtually eliminate the problems of acute toxic reactions.[49] Subdural placement is difficult to detect and requires vigilant ongoing clinical assessment and monitoring. Midwife top-ups should only be allowed if an anaesthetist is immediately available to attend the mother.[51]

A recommendation of the Standing Advisory Committee of the Royal College of Obstetricians and Gynaecologists was that 'Epidural analgesia should not be used unless a person capable of cardiopulmonary resuscitation (CPR) of the pregnant patient is present on the labour ward'. This was incorporated into the General Professional Training Guide of the College of Anaesthetists in 1987.[51]

Epidural infusions

A logical progression from the use of small increments of dilute solutions of local anaesthetic is the use of infusions of dilute doses as a safety measure to avoid the sudden changes that can occur with epidural top-ups.[51,53] Further experience is required with epidural infusions before their potential hazards can be fully evaluated; advantages include dispensing with midwife top-ups and uninterrupted analgesia. It has been found that for a given hourly dose, low concentration solutions are better than high concentrations.[54] Hicks *et al.*[55] found that infusion produced significantly better analgesia compared with bolus doses but no significant difference in motor block;

Flynn and colleagues[56] found that using weak solutions of local anaesthetic (0.08% compared with 0.25% at 20 m/hr), the plasma bupivacaine concentration was significantly lower, motor block was reduced but quality of analgesia unaffected. Jones and colleagues[57] in Cardiff found that midwives were very good at assessing the upper level of block during epidural infusions. They recommended that height of block should be assessed 2-hourly to avoid the block receeding too far before the next top-up, to detect inadvertent intrathecal infusion and to suspect the possibility of intravascular migration if the level of the block were falling.

Patient-controlled epidural analgesia

A further progression from epidural infusions is the use of PCEA. Advantages include patient control and the avoidance of delay between onset of pain and administration of analgesia. Disadvantages are that the equipment is bulky, expensive and can go wrong. Gambling et al.[58] compared bolus administration of 12 ml 0.125% bupivacaine with 1:400 000 adrenaline with PCEA of the same solution by 4 ml increments on demand with a limit of 12 ml/hr. Hourly bupivacaine requirements were virtually the same and produced similar sensory levels and pain relief in the two groups, although patient satisfaction was greater in the group using PCEA. Gambling and colleagues[59] compared 0.125% bupivacaine by continuous infusion 12 ml/hr (15 mg/hr) with PCEA infusion 4 ml/hr + 4 ml bolus on demand with a 20 minute lock-out period (i.e. 5–20 mg/hr). The patients in the PCEA group required less analgesia but the pain scores and height of sensory block were comparable.

Lysak et al.[60] found no significant advantage of PCEA over continuous epidural infusion but in that study the patients in the continuous infusion group were closely attended, topped up promptly as necessary and the infusion rate adjusted hourly. The addition of fentanyl 1 μg/ml to the epidural infusion mixture significantly reduces the hourly infusion requirement, and further addition of adrenaline produces a more dense block. A disadvantage of opioids is that they cause mild pruritus but this is usually a very minor problem elicited only on direct questioning. The advantage of PCEA is that the patient can titrate her own analgesia; this overcomes the great problem of variation in individual patient requirements during labour. Low basal infusion rates, small on-demand boluses and dilute local anaesthetic solutions all enhance PCEA safety. Any gradual dissipation of effect or increasing sensory level out of proportion to drug delivery should warn of intravascular or subarachnoid catheter migration respectively, before the development of deleterious effects. Every PCEA bolus functions as a partial subarachnoid test dose as the sensory level would increase abruptly. By programming a low hourly limit (20 ml 0.125% bupivacaine, 25 mg/hr), use of PCEA minimises the risk of systemic toxicity. Of the solutions tested to date, the low hourly infusion requirements and lack of significant adverse effects favour the use of a bupivacaine/fentanyl mixture for PCEA during labour. However, the wider application of PCEA during labour awaits large scale studies which will more fully describe the relative risks and benefits of this technique. Close patient monitoring is still of paramount importance.

The relative merits of currently available methods of epidural drug delivery for pain relief during labour have been reviewed by Brownridge.[61]

Withholding top-ups in the second stage is barbaric

Epidural opioids

In efforts to provide good second stage pain relief without increasing the incidence of instrumental delivery, there has been a move towards mixing opioids and bupivacaine during labour to provide good analgesia while avoiding unwanted motor blockade. Reynolds *et al.*[62] found that in patients with good T11–12 block but perineal pain in the first stage of labour, a combination of 100 µg fentanyl and 10 mg bupivacaine given epidurally produced good pain relief in all patients, while avoiding the concurrent motor effects of large doses of bupivacaine. Administration of methadone 5 mg epidurally prior to normal administration of bupivacaine 0.25% by bolus top-ups significantly reduced pain and motor blockade but did not significantly reduce bupivacaine requirements.[63] D'Athis *et al.*[64] found that an infusion of bupivacaine (25 mg/ml) with fentanyl (5 µg/ml) at 3 ml/hr provided better analgesia than the same mixture by intermittent top-ups with significantly lower dosage requirements. In a comparison of epidural bupivacaine infusion and bupivacaine with sufentanil infusion, Phillips[65] found that analgesia was significantly better in the group given the bupivacaine/sufentanil mixture, with fewer top-ups and less motor weakness. Brownridge[66] has reported that addition of 25 mg pethidine to 10 ml bupivacaine 0.125% epidural bolus top-ups provided analgesia of 75–90 minutes duration with absence of significant motor loss and shivering.

Chestnut and colleagues[67] found that maintenance of epidural infusion using a weak bupivacaine 0.0625%/fentanyl 0.0002% mixture during the second stage, compared to stopping the infusion at the end of the first stage, led to significantly better analgesia during the second stage in the treatment group with no significant increase in the incidence of instrumental delivery. 94% patients in the treatment group had no detectable motor block just before delivery compared with 100% patients in the non-treatment group. Naulty *et al.*[68] found an improvement in labour outcome as a result of continuing epidural analgesia during the second stage. This study retrospectively reviewed the labour records of patients before and after a change in epidural technique. The first group were given a loading dose of 1.5% ligno- caine with 1:200 000 adrenaline to attain a sensory block to T10, and then intermittent boluses of 1.5% lignocaine or 0.25%-0.5% bupiva- caine until full dilation. The second group were given 10 ml 0.25% bupivacaine with 5 μg/ml fentanyl initially and then 0.125%-0.25% bupivacaine with 2 μg/ml fentanyl until delivery. The change in tech- nique was associated with a significant increase in the percentage of patients receiving epidural analgesia for vaginal delivery and a significant decrease in the percentage of patients who eventually underwent LSCS or instrumental delivery.

Primiparae can be reassured that epidural analgesia does not increase the incidence of forceps delivery

Despite the fact that epidural analgesia does not appear to influence uterine activity in the first stage of labour, an analysis of uterine activity in spontaneous labour using a microcomputer[69] has shown a reduction in mean active pressure and contraction frequency and intensity during the second stage. Thus, although epidural analgesia has no effect on the length of the first stage of labour, it does prolong the second stage, and an infusion of oxytocin may be required to make good a relative deficiency.[70] Saunders *et al.*[71] have demonstrated that by using an oxytocin infusion during the second stage of labour in primiparous patients receiving epidural analgesia, it is possible to reduce the length of the second stage, the number of non-rotational forceps deliveries and the incidence of perineal trauma. It did not, however, decrease the number of rotational forceps deliveries for mal- position of the occiput. Johnsrud *et al.*[72] found that continuation of the epidural infusion 0.25% bupivacaine at 7 ml/hr (17.5 mg/hr) until delivery produced improved pain relief with no prolonged duration of the second stage when active management with syntocinon was commenced in the first stage following institution of effective epidural analgesia. There was no increase in the instrumental delivery rate even when the active pushing time was limited to one hour. The incidence of rotational forceps was lower than that in the control group.

Hicks *et al.*[55] compared the use of a continuous epidural infusion of 0.075% bupivacaine with the more conventional 0.5% bupivacaine top-ups for pain relief in labour. 51% of the top-up group had a spontaneous vaginal delivery as compared to 37% in the infusion group. The latter was also associated with a higher incidence of caesarean section, 19%, compared to 9% in the top-up group. There was no significant difference in the overall incidence of instrumental delivery between the groups.

Sadly we are still far from being in a position to reassure the primiparous woman of a spontaneous outcome of labour.

Epidural anaesthesia is contra-indicated in mothers on low-dose heparin

Institution of central conduction block regional anaesthesia (spinal or epidural) in obstetrical patients receiving low-dose ('mini') heparin prophylaxis remains as controversial today as it did when Dr E. Letsky and Dr J. Thorburn argued for and against its use, respectively, in the first volume. The concerns about the safety of combining low-dose heparin and epidural anaesthesia in the pregnant woman are based on lack of definitive data, theoretical grounds, and potential medicolegal implications.

The lack of definitive data remains as possibly the most common cause for this ongoing controversy, a fact highlighted by the absence of facts to enlighten us as to the correct management of this ever-increasing problem. The subject has been recently reviewed[73] but it is still true that there are no reported prospective controlled studies of complications from epidural anaesthesia in patients receiving low-dose heparin. The papers of Rao *et al.*[74] and Odoom *et al.*[75] remain as the largest retrospective studies of the decade.

The only mention in the literature in the past two years is a question posed by Russell,[76] a consultant urologist, who questioned the use of spinal anaesthesia in his urology patients many of whom were on low-dose heparin. Eichhorn *et al.* in reply advocate the safe use of the technique but highlight the need for evaluation of the patient's clotting status by checking the activated partial thromboplastin time to verify that there is no evidence of measurable systemic anticoagulation. Eichhorn in this respect confirms the arguments proposed by Dr Letsky, who described so successfully the theoretical basis for these laboratory tests in patients on low-dose heparin. Despite this, however, Darnet *et al.*[77] in their case report describe epidural haemotoma formation in a patient with an epidural catheter, despite normal activated partial thromboplastin time, prothrombin time and platelet count, receiving 12- hourly mini-dose heparin. This fact was the basis of the discussion by Parnass *et al.*[78] when replying to Eichhorn *et al.* These arguments serve to confirm the fact which Dr Thorburn drew to our attention namely the large interpatient variability and unpredicable response to low-dose heparin.

Although the absence of literature in relation to epidural anaesthesia and low-dose heparin is worthy of comment, it is also interesting to see the continued publications of case reports demonstrating the association between spinal epidural haemotoma and systemic heparinisation,[79,80,81] a fact well known and documented.

The main trend of research in the obstetric patient and coagulation abnormalities appears to remain within the forum of pre-eclampsia,[82,83] thrombocytopenia,[84,85] associated coagulation problems, and the theoretical use of coagulation studies in obstetric patients.[86] While this grey area also undoubtedly merits further research, it remains obvious that the question of the feasibility, both medically and medicolegally, of the clinical combination of low-dose heparin and epidural anaesthesia in the pregnant woman will remain unanswered until further prospective controlled studies help solve this important dilemma.

REFERENCES

1. Tordoff SG, Sweeney BP. Acid aspiration prophylaxis in 288 obstetric anaesthetic departments in the United Kingdom. *Anaesthesia* 1990; **45:** 776–80.
2. Burgess RW, Crowhurst JA. Acid aspiration prophylaxis in Australian obstetric hospitals—a survey. *Anaesthesia and Intensive Care* 1989; **17:** 492–5.
3. Ormezzano X, Francois TP, Viaud J-Y, Bukowski J-G, Bourgeonneau M-C, Cottron D, Ganansia M-F, Gregoire FM, Grinand MR, Wessel PE. Aspiration pneumonitis prophylaxis in obstetric anaesthesia: comparison of effervescent cimetidine–sodium citrate mixture and sodium citrate. *British Journal of Anaesthesia* 1990; **64:** 503–6.
4. Brock-Utne JG, Rout C, Moodley J, Mayat N. Influence of preoperative gastric aspiration on the volume and pH of gastric contents in obstetric patients undergoing caesarean section. *British Journal of Anaesthesia* 1989; **62:** 397–401.
5. Mathews HML, Moore J. Sodium bicarbonate as a single dose antacid in obstetric anaesthesia. *Anaesthesia* 1989; **44:** 590–1.
6. Gallagher EG, White M, Ward S, Cottrell J, Mann SG. Prophylaxis against acid aspiration syndrome. *Anaesthesia* 1988; **43:** 1011–4.
7. Escolano F, Castano J, Pares N, Bisbe E, Monterde J. Comparison of the effects of famotidine and ranitidine on gastric secretion in patients undergoing elective surgery. *Anaesthesia* 1989; **44:** 212–5.
8. Moote CA, Manninen PH. A random double-blind comparison of ranitidine and famotidine for acid aspiration prophylaxis in morbidly obese patients. *Canadian Journal of Anaesthesia* 1989; **36:** S143–4.
9. Moore J, Flynn RJ, Sampaio M, Wilson CM, Gillon KRW. Effect of single-dose omeprazole on intragastric acidity and volume during obstetric anaesthesia. *Anaesthesia* 1989; **44:** 559–62.
10. Gin T, Ewart MC, Yau G, Oh TE. Effect of oral omeprazole on intragastric pH and volume in women undergoing elective caesarean section. *British Journal of Anaesthesia* 1990; **65:** 616–9.
11. Ewart MC, Yau G, Gin T, Kotur CF, Oh TE. A comparison of the

effects of omeprazole and ranitidine on gastric secretion in women undergoing elective caesarean section. *Anaesthesia* 1990; **45:** 527–30.

12. Cruickshank RH, Morrison DA, Bamber PA, Nimmo WS. Effect of IV omeprazole on the pH and volume of gastric contents before surgery. *British Journal of Anaesthesia* 1989; **63:** 536–40.

13. Flynn RJ, Moore J, Collier PS, McClean E. Does pretreatment with cimetidine and ranitidine affect the disposition of bupivacaine? *British Journal of Anaesthesia* 1989; **62:** 87–91.

14. Flynn RJ, Moore J, Collier PS, Howard PJ. Single dose oral H$_2$-antagonists do not affect plasma lidocaine levels in the parturient. *Acta Anaesthesiologica Scandinavica* 1989; **33:** 593–6.

15. Dailey PA, Hughes SC, Rosen MA, Healy K, Cheek DBC, Shnider SM. Effect of cimetidine and ranitidine on lidocaine concentrations during epidural anesthesia for cesarean section. *Anesthesiology* 1988; **69:** 1013–7.

16. Flynn RJ, Moore J, Collier PS, Howard PJ. Effect of intravenous cimetidine on lignocaine disposition during extradural caesarean section. *Anaesthesia* 1989; **44:** 739–41.

17. O'Sullivan GM, Smith M, Morgan B, Brighouse D, Reynolds F. H$_2$ antagonists and bupivacaine clearance. *Anaesthesia* 1988; **43:** 93–5.

18. Kishikawa K, Namiki A, Miyashita K, Saitoh K. Effects of famotidine and cimetidine on plasma levels of epidurally administered lignocaine. *Anaesthesia* 1990; **45:** 719–21.

19. Raidoo DM, Marszalek A, Brock-Utne JG. Acid aspiration in primates (a surprising experimental result). *Anaesthesia and Analgesia* 1988; **16:** 375–6.

20. Raidoo DM, Rocke DA, Brock-Utne JG, Marszalek A, Engelbrecht HE. Critical volume for pulmonary acid aspiration: reappraisal in a primate model. *British Journal of Anaesthesia* 1990; **65:** 248–50.

21. Brown MA. Pregnancy induced hypertension: current concepts. *Anaesthesia and Intensive Care* 1989; **17:** 185–97.

22. Mudie LL, Lewis M. Pre-eclampsia: its anaesthetic implications. *British Journal of Hospital Medicine* 1990; **43:** 297–300.

23. Van Assche FA, Spitz B, Vansteelant L. Severe systemic hypertension during pregnancy. *American Journal of Cardiology* 1989; **63:** 22C-25C.

24. Duncan SLB. Does volume expansion in pre-eclampsia help or hinder? *British Journal of Obstetrics and Gynaecology* 1989; **96:** 631–3.

25. Graham SG, Luxton MC. The requirement for intensive care support for the pregnant population. *Anaesthesia* 1989; **44:** 581–4.

26. Clark SL, Cotton DB. Clinical indications for pulmonary artery catheterisation in the patient with severe pre-eclampsia. *American Journal of Obstetrics and Gynecology* 1988; **158:** 453–8.

27. Belfort M, Uys P, Dommisse J, Davey DA. Haemodynamic changes in gestational proteinuric hypertension: the effects of rapid volume expansion and vasodilator therapy. *British Journal of Obstetrics and Gynaecology* 1989; **96:** 634–41.

28. Kirshon B, Moise KJ, Cotton DB, Longmire S, Jones M, Tessem J, Joyce TA. Role of volume expansion in severe pre-eclampsia. *Surgery, Gynecology and Obstetrics* 1988; **167:** 367–71.

29.   Clark SL, Cotton DB. Clinical indications for pulmonary artery catheterization in the patient with severe pre-eclampsia. *American Journal of Obstetrics and Gynecology* 1988; **158:** 453–8.

30.   Cotton DB, Lee W, Huhta JC, Dorman KF. Hemodynamic profile of severe pregnancy-induced hypertension. *American Journal of Obstetrics and Gynecology* 1988; **158:** 523–9.

31.   Woodward DG, Romanoff ME. Is CVP monitoring 'contraindicated' in patients with severe pre-eclampsia? (letter) *American Journal of Obstetrics and Gynecology* 1989; **161:** 837–9.

32.   Baker AB. Management of severe pregnancy-induced hypertension, or gestosis, with sodium nitroprusside. *Anaesthesia and Intensive Care* 1990; **18:** 361–5.

33.   Kirshon B, Lee W, Mauer MB, Cotton DB. Effects of low-dose dopamine therapy in the oliguric patient with pre-eclampsia. *American Journal of Obstetrics and Gynecology* 1988; **159:** 604–7.

34.   Slater RM, Wilcox FL, Smith WD, Maresh MJA. Phenytoin in pre-eclampsia (letter). *Lancet* **2** (8673) 1224–5.

35a. Dinsdale HB. Does magnesium sulfate treat eclamptic seizures? Yes. *Archives of Neurology* 1988; **45:** 1360–1.

35b. Kaplan PW, Lesser RP, Fisher RS, Repke JT, Hanley DF. No, magnesium sulfate should not be used in treating eclamptic seizures. *Archives of Neurology* 1988; **45:** 1361–4.

36.   Hernandez C, Cunningham FG. Eclampsia. *Clinical Obstetrics and Gynaecology* 1990; **33:** 460–6.

37.   Pritchard JA. Magnesium sulphate in the treatment of eclampsia (letter). *Archives of Neurology* 1989; **46:** 947–8.

38.   Tuffnell D, O'Donovan P, Lilford RJ, Prys-Davies A, Thornton JG. Phenytoin in pre-eclampsia (letter). Lancet **2** (8673) 273–4.

39.   Harding DL, Leong CM. Intravenous clonazepam in eclampsia. *Australia and New Zealand Journal of Obstetrics and Gynaecology* 1988; **28:** 74–5.

40.   Silver HM. Acute hypertensive crisis in pregnancy. *Medical Clinics of North America* 1989; **73:** 623–38.

41.   Kaulhausen H, Wechsler E. Antihypertensive drug therapy during pregnancy. *Clinical and Experimental hypertension* 1988; **B7:** 213–25.

42.   Wasserstrum N, Kirshon B, Willis RS, Moise KJ, Cotton DB. Quantitative hemodynamic effects of acute volume expansion in severe pre-eclampsia. *Obstetrics and Gynecology* 1989; **73:** 546–50.

43.   Toppozada MK, Ismail AAA, Hegab HM, Kamel MA. Treatment of pre-eclampsia with prostaglandin A1. *American Journal of Obstetrics and Gynecology* 1988; **159:** 160–5.

44.   *Report on Confidential Enquiries into Maternal Deaths in the UK 1985–87.* London: HMSO, 1991.

45.   Scott DB. Editorial: test doses in extradural block. *British Journal of Anaesthesia* 1988; **61:** 129–30.

46.   Leighton BL, Norris MC, Sosis M, Epstein R, Chayen B, Larijani GE. Limitations of epinephrine as a marker of intravascular injection in laboring women. *Anesthesiology* 1987; **66:** 688–91.

47.   Sosis A, Scott DB, Thorburn J, Lim M. Limitations of adrenaline test

doses in obstetric patients undergoing extradural anaesthesia (letter). *British Journal of Anaesthesia* 1989; **62:** 578–9.

48. Selwyn Crawford J. Epidural test dose in obstetrics (letter). *Canadian Journal of Anaesthesia* 1988; **35** (4): 441–2.

49. Crowhurst JA, Burgess RW, Derham RJ. Monitoring epidural analgesia in the parturient. *Anaesthesia and Intensive Care* 1990; **18:** 308–13.

50. Prince GD, Shetty GR, Miles M. Safety and efficacy of a low volume extradural test dose of bupivacaine in labour. *British Journal of Anaesthesia* 1989; **62:** 503–8.

51. Morgan B. Unexpectedly extensive conduction blocks in obstetric epidural analgesia. *Anaesthesia* 1990; **45:** 148–52.

52. Van Zundert A, Vaes L, Soetens M, de Wolf A. Identification of inadvertent intravenous placement of an epidural catheter in obstetric anesthesia. *Anesthesiology* 1988; **68:** 142–5.

53. Lamont RF, Pinney D, Rodgers P, Bryant TN. Continuous versus intermittent epidural analgesia. *Anaesthesia* 1989; **44:** 893–6.

54. Richardson T. Epidural anaesthesia for obstetrics: where are we? *New Zealand Medical Journal* 1988; **101:** 657–8.

55. Hicks JA, Jenkins JG, Newton MC, Findley IL. Continuous epidural infusion of 0.075% bupivacaine for pain relief in labour. *Anaesthesia* 1988; **43:** 289–92.

56. Flynn RJ, McMurray TJ, Dwyer R, Moore J. Comparison of plasma bupivacaine concentrations during continuous extradural infusion in labour. *British Journal of Anaesthesia* 1988; **61:** 382–4.

57. Jones MJT, Bogod DG, Rees GAD, Rosen M. Midwives' assessment of the upper sensory level after epidural blockade. *Anaesthesia* 1988; **43:** 557–9.

58. Gambling DR, McMorland GH, Yu P, Laszlo C. Comparison of patient-controlled epidural analgesia and conventional 'top-up' injections during labor. *Anesthesia and Analgesia* 1990; **70:** 256–61.

59. Gambling DR, Yu P, Cole C, McMorland GH, Palmer L. A comparative study of patient controlled epidural analgesia (PCEA) and continuous infusion epidural analgesia (CIEA) during labour. *Canadian Journal of Anaesthesia* 1988; **35:** 249–54.

60. Lysak SZ, Eisenach JC, Dobson CE. Patient-controlled epidural analgesia during labor: a comparison of three solutions with a continuous infusion control. *Anesthesiology* 1990; **72:** 44–9.

61. Brownridge P. Epidural medication after the initial dose: reflections on current methods of administration during labour. *Anaesthesia and Intensive Care* 1990; **18:** 300–8.

62. Reynolds F, O'Sullivan G. Epidural fentanyl and perineal pain in labour. *Anaesthesia* 1989; **44:** 341–4.

63. Martin CS, McGrady EM, Colquhoun A, Thorburn J. Extradural methadone and bupivacaine in labour. *British Journal of Anaesthesia* 1990; **65:** 330–2.

64. D'Athis F, Macheboeuf M, Thomas H, Robert C, Desch G, Galtier M, Mares P, Eledjam JJ. Epidural analgesia with a bupivacaine-fentanyl mixture in obstetrics: comparison of repeated injections and continuous infusion. *Canadian Journal of Anaesthesia* 1988; **35:** 116–22.

65. Phillips G. Continuous infusion epidural analgesia in labor: the effect of adding sufentanil to 0.125% bupivacaine. *Anesthesia and Anelgesia* 1988; **67:** 462–5.

66. Brownridge P. Epidural bupivacaine-pethidine mixture; clinical experience using a low-dose combination in labour. *Australia and New Zealand Journal of Obstetrics and Gynaecology* 1988; **28:** 17–24.

67. Chestnut DH, Laszewski LJ, Pollack KL, Bates JN, Manago NK, Choi WW. Continuous epidural infusion of 0.0625% bupivacaine–0.0002% fentanyl during the second stage of labor. *Anesthesiology* 1990; **72:** 613–8.

68. Naulty JS, Smith R, Ross R. Effect of changes in labor analgesia practice on labor outcome. *Anesthesiology* 1988; **69:** A660.

69. Fairlie FM, Phillips GF, Andrews BJ, Calder AA. An analysis of uterine activity in spontaneous labour using a microcomputer. *British Journal of Obstetrics and Gynaecology* 1988; **95:** 57–64.

70. Reynolds F. Epidural analgesia in obstetrics: pros and cons for mother and baby. *British Medical Journal* 1989; **299:** 751–2.

71. Saunders NJStG, Spiby H, Gilbert L, Fraser RB, Hall JM, Mutton PM, Jackson A, Edmonds DK. Oxytocin infusion during second stage of labour in primiparous women using epidural analgesia: a randomised double blind placebo controlled trial. *British Medical Journal* 1989; **299:** 1423–6.

72. Johnsrud M-L, Dale PO, Lovland B. Benefits of continuous infusion epidural analgesia throughout vaginal delivery. *Acta Obstetrica Gynecologica Scandinavica* 1988; **67:** 355–8.

73. Stow PJ, Burrows FA. Anticoagulants in anaesthesia. *Canadian Journal of Anaesthasia* 1987; **34:** 632–49.

74. Rao TKO, El-Etr AA. Anticoagulation following placement of epidural and subarachnoid catheters. *Anesthesiology* 1981; **55:** 618–20.

75. Odoom JA, Sih IL. Epidural anaesthesia and anticoagulant therapy. *Anaesthesia* 1983; **38:** 254–9.

76. Russell D. Spinal anesthesia and anticoagulant. *Journal of the American Medical Association,* 1989; **262:** 411.

77. Darnet S, Guggiari M, Grob R, Guillaume A, Viars P. Lumbar epidural haematoma following the setting-up of an epidural catheter. *Ann Fr Anesth Reanim* 1986; **5:** 550–2.

78. Parnass SM, Rothenberg DM, Fischer RL, Ivankovich AD. Spinal anesthesia and mini-dose heparin. *Journal of the American Medical Association* 1990; **263:** 1496

79. Dickman CA, Shedd SA, Spetzler RF, Shjetter AG, Sonntag KH. Spinal epidural hematoma associated with epidural anesthesia: complications of systemic heparinization in patients receiving peripheral vascular thrombolytic therapy. *Anesthesiology* 1990; **72:** 947–50.

80. Messer HD, Forshan VR, Brust JCM, Hughes JEO. Transient paraplegia from hemotoma after lumbar puncture: a consequence of anticoagulant therapy. *Journal of the American Medical Association* 1976; **235:** 529–30.

81. Tekkok IH, Cataltepe O, Tahta K, Bertan V. Extradural haemotoma after continuous extradural anaesthesia. *British Journal of Anaesthesia* 1991; **67:** 112–15.

82. Schindler M, Gatt S, Isert P, Morgans D, Cheung A. Thrombocyto-penia and platelet functional defects in pre-eclampsia: implications for regional anaesthesia. *Anaesthesia and Intensive Care* 1990; **18:** 169–74.

83. Barker P, Callander CC. Coagulation screening before epidural anal-gesia in pre-eclampsia. *Anaesthesia* 1991; **46:** 64–7.

84. Burrows RF, Kelton JG. Thrombocytopenia at delivery: a prospective survey of 6715 deliveries. *American Journal of Obstetrics and Gynaecology* 1990; **162:** 731–4.

85. Hew-Wing P, Rolbin SH, Hew E, Amato D. Epidural anaesthesia and thrombocytopenia. *Anaesthesia* 1989; **44:** 775–7.

86. Basu S, Constantine G, Bareford D. The rational use of coagulation studies in obstetrics: an audit. *British Journal of Obstetrics and Gynaecology* 1990; **97:** 452–8.

Index